Counseling Persons with Communication Disorders and Their Families

Counseling Persons with Communication Disorders and Their Families

THIRD EDITION

David M. Luterman

pro·ed

8700 Shoal Creek Boulevard
Austin, Texas 78757-6897

pro·ed

©1996, 1991, 1984 by PRO-ED, Inc.
8700 Shoal Creek Boulevard
Austin, Texas 78757-6897

Library of Congress Cataloging-in-Publication Data

Luterman, David.
    Counseling persons with communication disorders and their families / David M. Luterman. — 3rd ed.
        p.   cm.
    Rev. ed. of: Counseling the communicatively disordered and their families. 2nd ed. 1991.
    Includes bibliographical references and index.
    ISBN 0-89079-680-7 (softcover : alk. paper)
    1. Communicative disorders—Patients—Counseling of.
2. Rehabilitation counseling.   I. Luterman, David.   Counseling the communicatively disordered and their families.   II. Title.
RC429.L87   1996
616.85′506—dc20   95-50274
                                        CIP

This book is designed in Berkeley Book.

Production Manager: Alan Grimes
Production Coordinator: Karen Swain
Managing Editor: Tracy Sergo
Art Director: Thomas Barkley
Reprints Buyer: Alicia Woods
Editor: Sue Motzer
Editorial Assistant: Claudette Landry
Editorial Assistant: Martin Wilson

Printed in the United States of America

3   4   5   6   7   8   9   10   00   99   98   97

To all clinicians who are
willing to learn from their clients

Contents

Foreword *ix*

Acknowledgments *xiii*

Introduction to the Third Edition *xv*

Introduction to the First Edition *xix*

Introduction to the Second Edition *xxiii*

1 Counseling by the Speech Pathologist and Audiologist *1*

2 Contemporary Theories of Counseling *9*

3 Erikson Life Cycle and Relationship *31*

4 The Emotions of Communication Disorders *47*

5 Counseling and the Diagnostic Process *75*

6 Techniques of Counseling *87*

7 The Group Process *111*

8 Working with Families *131*

9 Counseling and the Field of Communication Disorders *167*

References *179*

Index *189*

Foreword

The last decade has been witness to a revolution in the field of communication disorders. This revolution has been fueled by great advances in medical technology, computer applications, and "high-tech" instrumentation that have become essential tools in research and treatment of individuals with speech, language, and hearing impairments. In this third edition of *Counseling Persons with Communication Disorders and Their Families,* Dr. David M. Luterman makes the case that there also has been another, more quiet, more slowly moving revolution under way, which is certainly not as headline-grabbing and flashy as the technology revolution. The terms "raising of consciousness" and "gradual awakening" may more accurately reflect this increasing emphasis in communication disorders and other health-related fields—the awareness that treatment of persons and families with communication disorders should be, at its very core, a psychosocial process. David laments, however, that respect for the human service dimension of communication disorders has been slow in coming, and still takes a back seat to a focus on technique and fact-oriented education and training of our students.

David was an early torchbearer of the humanistic and family-centered emphasis in communication disorders, and in this third edition, he once again persuasively argues that a clinician in communication disorders must be as skilled in working with and supporting people as in applying specific speech–language or audiological assessment or therapy techniques. Furthermore, David clearly communicates that to be an effective clinician, simply having good intentions, or being able to empathize with persons and families challenged by a communication disorder, is not good enough. A clinician must have working knowledge of how a disability impacts a client and family, and how people generate their own capacities and strategies for coping (both adaptive and maladaptive) under what can be extremely stressful and challenging circumstances.

It is David's respect for the intricacy and complexity of the counseling process that makes his message so special. The prevailing attitude in many health-related professions is that supporting and counseling families is the easy part of the work and should not require special training. After all, we are in this profession because we care about people! Yet, to this day, I continue to be astonished by the "war stories" I hear from families about how the educational or health care system and its professionals (who probably consider themselves well-intentioned and sensitive clinicians) cause as much or greater stress for the family than the disability itself. Furthermore, when clinicians and students discuss the aspect of their work that is most challenging and therefore the source of most professional discomfort and anxiety, working with families and clients around emotional issues such as coping with a disability is invariably at the top of the list. Clearly, we can do much better in working with clients and in training our students.

And this is the message that David infuses throughout this book. David's philosophy of counseling is, at its very core, deeply rooted in an optimistic belief in human capacity for growth and change. Consistent with his philosophy, this book does not focus on the "affected patient"— the capacity for growth is an issue for systems of human relationships; that is, for professionals, clients, and their families, as well as for students in training. For persons and families affected by a disability, David believes that adaptation and coping is largely a process of making meaning out of difficult circumstances, and through this process, finding opportunities for individual and family growth. Because persons and families are so different by virtue of family structure, culture and religion, and specific circumstances surrounding the disability, by necessity, this process is highly subjective and individual. David contends that with the support and guidance of a trained clinician (when needed), the ultimate outcome for a person or family may include empowerment in advocacy and decision making, a greater sense of confidence in coping with challenges, more fulfilling relationships within the family, and in some cases, a reconsideration of one's life path. According to David, a belief in the basic competence of families must underlie the counseling process. For it is with this belief that families can be supported in making (and owning) the most important decisions regarding the affected person and other family members.

This same philosophy is the foundation of David's practices in training professionals in communication disorders and other health-related professions. That is, for effective counseling, the learning of techniques and facts is pointless without the development of a self-generated philosophy consonant with one's own belief system. Thus, David contends that students and professionals need to be able to make mistakes, learn from them, and not be afraid to feel the pain of their clients. The role of mentors and supervisors is to listen, support, and guide, but not to provide prescriptions and the "right" answers. It is through this process that students and professionals come to understand and accept their own personal and professional vulnerability, and ultimately, to better understand those whom they serve. David argues that this process allows clinicians to discard professional masks and scripts in order to truly be able to support the individual and unique human needs of our clients. I have observed that some clinicians may eventually reach this level of "expertise" through years of professional and personal experience. However, as David accurately points out, professional training and constraints inherent in work settings may actually impede such development and encourage a detached working demeanor. Fortunately, through David's writings, readers will benefit from the lessons learned from his long and distinguished career as a clinician and professor, as well as his own and his family's personal challenges.

For the professional and student, this book is, in part, about taking risks. The risks include reflecting deeply about how we relate to our clients and their families, and whether we take the more difficult path of understanding their pain and grief or remain objectively detached. The risks also include immersing ourselves in a world where simple prescriptions do not work and where there are no cut-and-dried answers. Yet, if we must avoid a "cookbook" approach, we must still be able to move forward and be effective in our relationships with clients and their families. The ultimate risk is to care too much about our life's work and the persons who receive our services. But with these risks comes the greatest reward—the sense that working with clients with communication disorders and their families is an integrated part of our lives, and part of our human growth and development, rather than simply a vocation that pays the bills.

For those students and professionals ready to take on these risks in the interest of their own professional and personal growth, I can think of no greater mentor than Dr. David M. Luterman. Largely due to the last four years of David's mentorship and friendship, I have grown tremendously in my understanding, and therefore, in my effectiveness in working with clients and families, and with my students. Although I have worked closely with children and families for many years (with the assumption that I was a good clinician), I now experience a challenge and depth in my work that far exceeds what I knew in the past. Those of us who have been able learn directly from David have been very fortunate. It is my sincerest wish that you who read this book also are ready to be nourished by the wisdom and experience that David offers, for I am confident that you, too, will experience greater fulfillment and challenge in your work.

In the Introduction to the second edition of this book, David stated that he would be content if his epitaph read, "He expanded our field by directing our attention to feelings and families." With this third edition, I can respond, "He continues to do so, and with great eloquence."

Barry M. Prizant, PHD, CCC-SLP
Division of Communication Disorders
Emerson College

Acknowledgments

I have yet to join the twentieth century, let alone the rapidly approaching twenty-first century. I write all my books at my kitchen table using a ballpoint pen (my wife made me give up my quill and ink) on yellow lined legal paper. Consequently I am in dire need of a skilled typist: one who can read my scrawl and use a word processor. Fortunately I have found such a one in Chris Starratt, who is able to do all of that and remain cheerful and calm to boot. I owe her a debt of gratitude. I am ever grateful to the support of the Administration of Emerson College, which granted me a sabbatical to write this third edition and provided me with the institutional support necessary for me to complete the work. Liz Bezera, librarian par excellence, was extremely helpful in obtaining references for me. And as always, I am grateful to my wife, Cari, who is so supportive of all my endeavors.

Introduction to
the Third Edition

I t is time to pick up my pen again, perhaps for the last time, prompted in large part by the recent article in *ASHA* by Culpepper, Mendel, and McCarthy (1994), which indicated that there has been little change in the number of counseling courses within our training programs since their last survey eight years ago. A computer search of our literature also indicates almost nothing new on counseling issues, yet almost everyone in training programs, according to Culpepper et al. (1994), believes that counseling is an important component of effective therapy and should be basic to the training of clinicians. It seems that counseling for us as a profession is much like Mark Twain's quip about the weather: Everybody talks about it but nobody does anything about it. I have long suspected that the reason for the dearth of literature and coursework is the lack of experienced teachers within our profession who have the dual knowledge of counseling process and communication disorders. The majority of our programs that offer a counseling course still offer it as a nondepartmental elective (Culpepper, 1994). This indicates to me that we don't have the teachers within our profession who have the requisite skills and knowledge.

One of my major justifications for writing this new edition is to make the text more teacher friendly in the hope that more instructors will be emboldened to adopt this text and offer a counseling course. In keeping with this rationale, I have also written a manual for teaching a course in counseling; this manual is available from the publisher. And, if teachers don't offer a specific course, I hope they will infuse their communication disorders curriculum with counseling notions. Since the last edition of this text, I have been in contact with several instructors at other universities who are trying to teach counseling. Many of them have been teaching from a technique orientation, using role-playing class activities and detailing therapists' responses to specific client situations. I think trying to teach counseling from a technique orientation is counterproductive. It is easy to teach this way, and students are happy because it gives them a structure to hold on to; however, approaching counseling from a technique orientation reduces the naturalness of the interpersonal encounter, which is, I believe, the heart of good counseling. Students with a technique orientation are left self-conscious and mechanical in their responses to client feelings. Good counseling needs to be seamless, and the process must be natural to the personality of the clinician. I am reminded of the story of the annual golf tournament that was held in a small town. Each year one man would beat out another until the second place finisher gave the winner a book entitled "How to Play Golf." After that he won every year.

I have been teaching a counseling course at Emerson College for the past 15 years and I have also taught intensive counseling courses at several universities. I am convinced that the most fruitful way to teach counseling is through a personal growth paradigm. The course itself needs to be a genuine encounter between the instructor and students to encourage personal growth of the students. In short, the instructor is always modeling good counseling interaction by using the students' life experiences as the raw material for learning. To be sure, there is a body of cognitive material that needs to be learned. At the least, our students need to be exposed to it, and I have left intact in this edition all cognitive material from previous editions, adding to it where appropriate.

The content and the specifics of counseling technique, however, should not be the major focus of the course. Effective counseling (and good therapy) is basically a right-brain experience. We need to be able to operate from our intuitive center. Too often our teaching is of the left-brain variety, whereby we teach students academic performance without clinical competency. Very often it isn't until students let go of what they have learned in school that they become truly effective clinicians. Our goal as educators must be to give students a solid knowledge base that is integrated with and guided by their clinical intuitions and feelings. We must give our students permission to be authentic human beings in a genuine encounter with their clients. The dilemma for the teacher is how to balance right- and left-brain teaching. I hope this edition of the text will provide help for the instructor in doing just that.

I have also finally completed writing the book describing my family's struggle with multiple sclerosis (*In the Shadows: Living and Coping with a Loved One's Chronic Illness,* 1995). This book was a long time in the writing (nearly 10 years) as I kept putting it aside to work on other projects. The writing for me was also very painful; the story was ever changing as we moved and are moving further down the disability path. In writing that book I delved deeply into the disability literature and how chronic illness of a significant adult affects families. This hard-won information is now incorporated into a very much revised Chapter 8. In the previous edition, that chapter was very much skewed to the families with young children with disabilities; it is now in better balance.

What I have come to realize in an increasing way is how important the marriage is—whether it be spousal or parental—to the eventual success of our clients. Working with families of newly diagnosed deaf children has shown me that the children who turn out best are the products of a strong marriage; I have also found that the adults with disabilities who are coping most successfully are the ones with strong marriages. In the third edition, especially in the revised chapter on families, I have addressed marriage as a key component of successful coping for our clients.

Once again, several gurus have influenced me strongly through their books: Gardner's (1991) book, *The Unschooled Mind*, in which he makes a strong case for experiential learning, has influenced my thinking about how best to teach counseling. Nuland's (1994) book, *How We Die*, and Levine's (1982) book, *Who Dies*, have reinforced for me again the notion of how time limited we all are and therefore how fragile and precious life is. These notions are vital to the success of the counselor. Levine's (1979) other book, *A Gradual Awakening*, has helped me learn to meditate and find the centering calm that enables me to listen, which I believe is the essence of good counseling. I have recently begun to bring meditation into the classroom with generally favorable reactions from the students.

My preoccupation with death is not morbid, but living with death awareness for me means that I do not postpone living; my wife's illness has also taught me that. Recently, I passed my 60th birthday, and the inexorable progression of my wife's illness and her increasing disability have restricted the time and energy I can devote to professional endeavors. I can sense the closing down of my very active involvement in professional affairs. I hope to continue teaching and doing occasional workshops, and it is my fondest wish that this text should become the stimulus for the creation of more counseling courses in our field that are taught by instructors with a background in communication disorders.

Introduction to
the First Edition

More than 20 years ago I started my career as a clinical audiologist. At that time I thought I was interested in the precision and surety that working with machines seemed to give. I soon realized that I was not a "machine person" but rather a "people person" and that the audiologic machinery was getting in the way of my relating to people. It was with some trepidation that I decided to come out from behind my audiometer and relate as a person rather than as a professional. The first outward manifestation of my slowly evolving inner changes was the willingness to wear nonwhite shirts; soon I went tieless. A few years later, I abandoned suits and sports jackets—the uniform of the male professional. Most recently I have given up all titles and prefer people to call me by my first name. These changes took more than 10 years to accomplish.

Rather than make a radical change in my life, I sought another way of relating to the hearing-impaired population. It became apparent to me that parents of severely hearing-impaired children were not being treated well. I was the clinical audiologist who confirmed the parents' suspicion that they had a deaf child, who proceeded to talk extensively about a course of action, and who then referred them to an educational facility. My information giving was designed to keep me in control of the situation, to conform to the parents' expectations and my own perception of what a professional was, and to distance the parents from their feelings, which I did not know how to handle. It also became apparent to me, on subsequent visits, that the needs of parents were not being met by either the educational facilities or by me. So with a great deal of naivete, I decided in 1965 to begin a parent-centered nursery program at Emerson College in Boston. In addition to a nursery and language therapy for the children, the Emerson program provided a once-a-week session designed as a parent support group, which I led. I decided early to forego my information-providing function (I had to—I had only a small number of set speeches and I was committing myself to 30 sessions with the parents) and spent much of each session listening to the parents. The program has continued to the present day and has afforded me a great opportunity to grow both personally and professionally. Out of my experience came a book describing the program in detail with procedures for counseling parents of hearing-impaired children (Luterman, 1979).

I found as I allowed more affect (feelings) to enter into these relationships (I could, for example, allow the parents to cry), listened more, and dealt less with content, that people learned more. When the information was spaced over time, and when I allowed parents to work through their very normal feelings about having a deaf child, the parents could absorb and retain the information I was providing. I realized in my audiologist mode that all those brilliant set speeches that I had been delivering had not been retained by the parents anyway, as on subsequent visits I found that parents were asking me questions that I thought I had already covered adequately. I also discovered that people were not as fragile as I had thought (actually, it was my own fragility I had been worrying about) and that they could defend themselves quite well against my insensitivities and all-too-frequent lack of skill. As long as I remained a caring, listening person, growth occurred within the relationship. I seemed to serve parents much better when I did not function in the traditional information-providing mode. As an added bonus I found that my professional boredom was replaced by excitement.

During the past several years, I have been teaching courses and giving workshops on counseling issues to working audiologists and speech pathologists. These experiences have made me aware that attitudes have not changed very much regarding counseling in the 20-odd years since I started working as a professional. Counseling as practiced by most audiologists and speech–language pathologists still seems to be of the information-imparting or advice-giving variety (i.e., the medical or quasimedical model). If the relationship between the professional and the individual with communication disorders gets into the emotional area, the audiologist/speech–language pathologist becomes uncomfortable and tends to hide behind content or to refer the patient to a social worker or psychologist. The information-providing role, however, is not satisfactory over the long run. One is apt to be bored delivering all the set speeches accumulated over a working lifetime. Professionals dealing with communication disorders who wish to change tend, after a few years of information providing, to seek other ways of relating to those they are helping; hence the attendance at workshops on counseling.

Those professionals who do not find another way of relating tend to "burn out" quickly. The burnout rate in our field is quite high; 43% of surveyed speech pathologists reported moderate to severe burnout, which involved a loss of concern for the feelings of their clients (Miller & Potter, 1982).

I think it is generally acknowledged that counseling skills are an important concomitant of the well-trained speech pathologist, yet little formal training is provided in educational programs. An examination of graduate catalogs indicates few courses offered specifically on counseling for the speech clinician, nor is a course in counseling required for certification by the American Speech-Language-Hearing Association.

Counseling skills, when they are obtained by graduate clinicians, seem to be obtained informally through students' observation of other clinicians or almost incidentally picked up as students acquire specific skills in altering speech and language behavior. Too many of our students are leaving training programs with a very limited view of their capacity to involve themselves in intensive relationships with their clients.

This book was initiated—as I suspect many texts are—when I agreed to teach a course on counseling the communicatively disordered and found that there was no single, satisfactory text. The ultimate purpose of this book is to demystify the counseling experience for the professional working within the field of communication disorders. It is my hope that as a result of reading this book, clinicians will feel more comfortable in allowing the affect that is a normal concomitant of having a communication disorder to emerge in their clinical interactions. I hope this book will provide some insight into relationship building and how it affects the counseling process. By allowing more affect to occur in the relationships, speech–language pathologists and audiologists will find that their information-providing role will be enhanced and they will therefore be much more effective. I think they will also obtain more job satisfaction.

This text is not intended to supplant the clinical use of social workers or psychologists: they are trained professionals whose skills will be needed within a comprehensive speech–language and hearing program. I hope, however, that this text will lead to a modified use of professional counselors so that they can provide support and ongoing inservice training to speech pathologists/audiologists as they deal with the normal emotions surrounding a communication disorder and provide direct service to emotionally disordered clients who may also have a communication disorder.

During the past several years I have come to value highly the use of Erik Erikson's stages of growth as a means of understanding both the difficulties of the communicatively disordered and the development of a counseling relationship. Recently I have come across the writings of Irvin Yalom on existential issues in psychotherapy, which I believe have far-reaching implications for the field of communication disorders. This text reflects my expanded appreciation of both Yalom and Erikson.

I have devoted a chapter to group counseling, as I feel that this area of counseling can be better utilized by the speech and hearing clinician. I have also devoted more space to the denial mechanism than I did in my previous book because I have come to see more clearly how the difficulties of the professional in handling the complex issue of denial limit effective counseling.

In writing this book I have drawn heavily on my own experience in the field of deafness and, in particular, on my work with parents. I have made no attempt to delineate content counseling for the specific speech disorders as I assume that the well-trained speech–language pathologist has this information. Once the professional acquires counseling skills, they are applicable to all disorders. By extension, much of the material is also appropriate for other disabling conditions, which do not necessarily involve a communication disorder. I hope that this book is of use to any professional working with the communicatively disordered who wishes to get beyond the information-providing role.

Introduction to the Second Edition

An author never really knows when a book is finished: A bell doesn't go off and nobody taps you on the shoulder. More often than not you are just exhausted and fed up with the material. (Apollinaire said, "Novels are never finished; they are only abandoned.") Such was the case with the first edition of this book. I had just felt written out, although I knew as I was writing the chapter on the family that here was a rich lode of material that needed to be mined at a later date. The material on family led me into literature seldom utilized in our field and subsequently became the book *Deafness in the Family* (1987).

During the intervening years since the publication of the first edition, my wife Cari developed multiple sclerosis. We actually knew she had it at the time I was writing the first edition of this book, but it was relatively benign and was not really interfering with our very busy lives. Five years after the publication of the first edition, the disease had progressed to the point where it was and has become a very important and dominating factor in our lives. This prompted me to look at how people, especially the well family members, can cope with chronic, progressive illness of a loved one; it was a study of powerlessness—in the face of diseases such as multiple sclerosis, Alzheimer's disease, arthritis, lupus, and diabetes. This study became the as-yet unpublished manuscript *The Shadow People*. This study brought me outside the field of communication disorders and made me realize again how universal the counseling and coping issues are.

My experiences in writing these two more recent books after completing the first edition of this book gave me much more material that needed to be incorporated into the second edition of this book.

In addition, several studies have been published since the first edition, notably the studies of Martin, George, O'Neal, and Daly (1987) and Williams and Derbyshire (1982), which indicate that audiologists in particular were ineffective in their counseling (although I suspect that if the same studies were done with speech pathologists, similar results would occur). The need for counseling skills in our profession is almost self-evident, yet somehow we are still failing to train students effectively in these counseling skills. McCarthy, Culpepper, and Lucks (1986), in their survey of departmental chairs, found that only 12% of the respondents felt that training programs were effective in training students in counseling. As a consequence of our ineptitude, many functioning clinicians are bereft of good counseling abilities and are, therefore, not very effective in what they do.

Counseling cuts across all disorders—it is both universal and timeless, based as it is on good interpersonal relationships. Once we get away from disorder-specific and content-based thinking, we can see the commonality of our universe. Under the disability skin we are all brothers and sisters, and it makes no difference whether we counsel stutterers, parents of deaf children, aphasics, or well family members of chronically ill people. We are dealing with loss, and the grief response seems universal in our culture. Grieving people need to be in a relationship with a responsive and caring professional who is equipped with good counseling skills.

As stated in the introduction to the first edition and which bears repeating here, it is not the purpose of this book to make "counselors" of speech pathologists and audiologists—to supplant the work of social workers or psychologists in a clinical setting. Rather it is to help the professionals who work with the communicatively disordered to incorporate some of the knowledge and skills of trained counselors in order to enhance their own clinical effectiveness. In short, the purpose is to make us clinicians as opposed to technicians, to move us beyond the narrow technical base of our field into a much more expansive one that allows and encourages speech pathologists and audiologists to work with and be comfortable about the myriad of feelings that accompany a communication disorder. We are working with people who are emotionally upset, not necessarily emotionally disordered and, as such, we need to develop the skills to deal with emotional adjustment issues and family issues.

I also would like to draw attention to the well family members. When there is a communication disorder in a family, everyone is affected by it, and it therefore becomes the responsibility of the speech pathologist and the audiologist to work with the needs of all members of the family.

A communication disorder always exists within a "family" context. It cannot be confined to a single individual because the disorder manifests itself only within the milieu of a relationship. For us to be effective, to be clinicians, we must examine and deal with the whole relationship. I have found in my professional life by working intimately with parents of deaf children, if you take good care of the parents, the children will do well. This admonition applies equally well to the chronically ill; if you take good care of the spouse and other family members, the identified patient also will do well. Failure to deal with family needs almost invariably limits therapeutic effectiveness. In this text "client" refers as much to the family member as it does to the identified person with a communication disorder.

When my professional epitaph gets written, and I hope it is not yet for a while, I would like it to say, "He expanded our field by directing our attention to feelings and families." In this new edition, which I hope will appeal to both the student in training and the practicing clinician, the reader will find the following changes:

Chapter 1 is an entirely new chapter reflecting the literature of our ineffectiveness as counselors and presenting my own definition and model of counseling.

Chapter 2 on contemporary theories of counseling is a compilation of material that is in the first edition. My love affair with existentialism and its application to our field continues unabated. I still value humanism very highly, and I have a grudging respect for the potent contributions that behaviorism and the rational/emotive approaches can make in our field.

Chapter 3 is the only chapter unchanged from the first edition. I think Erikson's life cycle model is such a powerful and universal tool that students and clinicians need to be exposed to it. It is also very useful for understanding relationship building.

Chapter 4 on the emotions is material that was scattered throughout the first edition. In this chapter the material has been rewritten and recast to reflect how emotions can lead to self-defeating behavior and, if not handled well by the clinicians, can undermine any effective therapy. In particular, it is the nonunderstanding of the denial mechanism and its role in the coping process by us as a profession that limits our effectiveness.

Chapter 4 also contains new material on coping that reflects my research with the families of the chronically ill. Here the clinician will find a model of the coping process and techniques for coping that can be applied to a broad clinical caseload.

Chapter 5 on the diagnostic process is a new one, and reflects my increasing awareness of the importance of the imprinting that occurs in the initial contact between clients and professionals. The diagnostic process can be and should be handled in such a way as to minimize the denial mechanism and to facilitate all subsequent client/professional interactions.

Chapter 6 on the techniques of counseling is an expanded chapter that gives more material for the clinician to practice effective listening, as well as suggestions for reframing which I am increasingly seeing as a very useful clinical intervention when used judiciously. I am also including "hypothetical" families in this chapter. This was a technique that I used and wrote about in my very first book. I think this can be a useful "case study" approach for beginning clinicians, as well as a technique to stimulate and direct group discussion.

Chapter 7 on the group process is slightly expanded from the first edition. I stand very committed to the group process as a strong healing and educational vehicle. I want very much to encourage and support the development of more groups within our field. To this end we need to develop competence and confidence in group facilitating. I ardently hope this chapter does both.

Chapter 8 on the family is completely rewritten and markedly expanded, reflecting material that was in *Deafness in the Family.* In particular, I think the material on the optimal and the successful families will be of use to the practicing clinician.

Chapter 9 is my attempt to look ahead for our field and to see how counseling skills will enrich our growth as a profession and in training students.

It is now time for me to "abandon" this manuscript. I think I have shared all I know at this point, and although nobody is tapping me on the shoulder and no bells are going off, I know it is time for me to stop. At this point I feel good that this volume accurately reflects my 30 years of clinical and teaching experience.

1

Counseling by the Speech Pathologist and Audiologist

As an aspiring audiologist in training, I learned that counseling was something one did after obtaining a careful case history and administering the diagnostic tests. Counseling was always information based and involved an explanation of the audiogram and recommendations for follow-through. I don't recall if the graduate students were given an explicit injunction not to deal with the client's feelings, but we behaved as though we were. If a client displayed feelings (e.g., by crying), we were to refer the client to the clinical psychologist. The message I received in my training program was that client affect was the province of social workers and psychologists and that counseling by audiologists and speech pathologists was to be information based. This was essentially a medical model of counseling and reflected, I think, a desire to keep the field of communication disorders as a distinct entity as well as to avoid infringing on other professions. It also, I think, reflected the lack of training in counseling in graduate programs at that time. Additionally, staying with content was professionally safe: With content, students could control the interactions; emotions were unpredictable and therefore potentially disruptive. With the medical model, students could adopt an attitude of detached concern and proceed to control the clinical interaction by delivering set speeches.

The medical model, at least among audiologists, remains the prevalent counseling approach. Flahive and White (1982), in a questionnaire

1

study of 226 audiologists, found that a great proportion of their time was spent in informational counseling as opposed to personal adjustment counseling. The audiologists also reported that in their training programs they had been exposed to much more informational counseling (90%) than personal adjustment counseling (10%).

Many audiologists and speech pathologists receive no training in counseling. McCarthy et al. (1986) surveyed training programs accredited by the American Speech-Language-Hearing Association. They found that only 40% of the programs offered a course in counseling within the department (36% had an out-of-department course and 23% had no offering at all). The most telling finding was that although the overwhelming majority of respondents felt that counseling was an important skill for speech pathologists to acquire, only 12% of the respondents felt that training programs were effective in training students in counseling. As noted in the Introduction to this book, a repeat of this survey (Culpepper et al., 1994) indicates little change in the number of counseling courses offered in our training programs.

The lack of training is reflected in an increasing body of information indicating that audiologists are not effective in their counseling. Williams and Derbyshire (1982) questioned 25 parents of children with severe and profound hearing impairment under the age of 11 within one year of their having been seen by an audiologist. The results of the questionnaire study and personal interviews are startling and rather disheartening. The responses indicated that 84% of the parents were unable to understand all of the information they had been given, 72% did not know what a hearing loss would mean to their children, and 64% did not have a realistic appreciation of how hearing loss would affect their own lives. When asked by the investigators to restate the audiologist's explanations of the implications of hearing loss, 40% could not do so at all and 24% attempted explanations that the investigators felt were incorrect. Martin, Krueger, and Bernstein (1990) conducted a questionnaire survey of 35 adults with hearing impairment shortly after they had had an audiological examination and had received content counseling from the audiologist. The authors concluded that "even when audiologists feel they have adequately covered all of the information during the audiological examination, the hearing-impaired adults' knowledge of this information is still lacking" (p. 32). Incredibly, not one respondent in their survey knew what an "audiogram" was after having just completed the examination.

In a national survey of audiologists and parents of children with hearing impairment, Martin et al. (1987) found that there were many important dissimilarities in the perceptions of audiologists and parents, primary among which were the differences in acceptance of deafness and in who should provide the counseling.

In an unpublished master's thesis, Lerner (1988) interviewed in depth the parents of a young deaf child (diagnosed at age two months) and the audiologists who had tested the child and counseled the parents. The parents were sophisticated, the father a physician and the mother a computer programmer. The audiologists were very experienced, both with doctoral degrees and 10 to 12 years of experience. The audiologists felt that they had done a good job of conveying the necessary information. The parents, on the other hand, were very dissatisfied, feeling that jargon was inappropriately used. For example, they felt the term "severe to profound" in describing their child's hearing loss was useless to them. (How often do audiologists use that terminology so casually?) What the parents most remembered was the tone of the comments, which to them was negative and pessimistic.

In my own clinical experience, this reaction is fairly typical of parents of newly diagnosed deaf children. When they leave the audiologists, they feel very confused and emotionally hurt and have not absorbed much of the informational counseling provided. Parents invariably remember irrelevant details—the dress the audiologist was wearing or the color of a tie—and although they retain little content, they always remember the emotional tone set by the audiologist—whether he or she was upbeat, hopeful, and emotionally supportive, or cold and factual.

Perhaps the crowning blow to our counseling egos was delivered by the study of Haas and Crowley (1982). The results of their survey indicated that parents of deaf children felt that the professional who provided them with the most meaningful information was the educator rather than the audiologist.

Certainly, some effective counseling is being provided within our field, and at times providing information is very appropriate. The audiologists in the Lerner (1988) study did have many successes; at the same time, however, we can be more effective as a profession if we are sensitive to the emotional state of our clients and feel comfortable in allowing affect to be a component of our clinical interactions.

It would seem that I am picking on the counseling skills of audiologists since all of the previous studies detailing failure of counseling were related to hearing disorders. Unfortunately, there are no comparable studies in speech pathology. These studies badly need to be done. I suspect they will yield comparable results if the information provided by speech–language pathologists is offered without recourse or sensitivity to the emotional state of the client.

In addition to counseling by informing, many professionals in our field counsel by persuading, which is a very seductive model of counseling. The underlying assumption of this approach is that "I as a professional have all of this information and experience. You as the client are ignorant of so many things that you need to know; therefore, I can make a better decision for you than you can for yourself." This approach often confirms clients' perceptions of their own limitations; they generally are feeling so inadequate and overwhelmed by the problem at hand that they often acquiesce to our arguments and recommendations and let the "doctor" decide. This is particularly true in the counseling of hearing parents of deaf children. A blatant example of counseling by persuasion can be found in an article by Dee (1981), in which she describes her total communication program for parents of children with hearing impairment. (It could just as well have been an oral program. The issue here is the counseling style, not the methodology.)

The role of parent education in developing and sustaining positive attitudes towards total communication.

Most hearing parents of deaf infants need considerable help and guidance in developing clear and honest convictions about the real values of the total communication approach in the life of a deaf infant and his/her family. Even after their first pleasurable experience with total communication, during family sessions, when they have learned to use the simultaneous method to achieve a warm and loving communicative interaction with their infant, some of our parents will continue to undergo periods of doubt, uncertainty and even occasional resistance. Parents might also be struggling against non-supportive and/or antagonistic attitudes toward manual communication expressed by grandparents, relatives and friends. Furthermore, almost all parents cannot help but be vulnerable to the highly persuasive claims of the oralist. It is essential, therefore, to provide parents in total communication programs with a strong and convincing rationale for continuing to use this communication mode. A parent education program can provide year-long opportunities for exploring and evaluating all that is 'total' about total communication and for expanding and strengthening parental understanding of and belief in the emotional and educational gains that are the rewards of a total communication way of life. (p. 15)

This mode of counseling assumes that parents are weak and are incapable of effective decision making: People generally conform to our expectations of them.

I, too, can recall persuading clients. A druggist with a very significant hearing loss once came in with his wife because she had been nagging him to get a hearing aid. Both the wife and I ganged up on him to persuade him to get an aid; she was arguing about how hard it was to live with him and I was arguing about how difficult it must be at work and how hazardous it might be for his customers. He finally agreed to get the aid, but a follow-up call 6 months later indicated that the hearing aid was in the drawer most of the time and the wife was as frustrated and angry as ever.

Counseling by persuasion is almost always a poor approach because the clients never "own" their behavior. They do not take responsibility for having made the decision. The responsibility remains with the professional. My own experience in deafness has been that parents who have been persuaded to sign with their children are the ones who drop out of sign class early and seldom use total communication at home; likewise, clients who are persuaded to get a hearing aid seldom wear it on a regular basis. True change comes from the inside: The person has made a decision and is willing to commit to it.

The second problem with counseling by persuasion is that it reinforces the client's feelings of inadequacy. It becomes a confirmation of his or her own felt inability to make a good decision, and therefore the decision is to "trust the professional." This creates the dependent client—the one who is less apt to take any initiatives or responsibilities for solving the problem. The work is all left to the speech pathologist or audiologist who "knows better." This situation also tends to create the fanatic parents—those who have been "brainwashed" and must now believe ardently in a particular approach, which has to be right because they have no other recourse, not having developed any confidence in themselves or in their decision-making skills. These are parents who do not think reflectively—they just believe. This is neither good education nor good counseling.

The two counseling approaches—counseling by informing and counseling by persuading—are not mutually exclusive. There are components of both in most counseling sessions. After first informing the client of test results, we often set about convincing him or her of what to do about the data. A combination of informing and persuading counseling strategies can be very potent. When we overwhelm with information, we also undermine the client's confidence, leaving him or her very vulnerable to being persuaded.

A third approach to counseling clients is one I prefer: counseling by listening and valuing. In this approach, the clients are seen as possessing the wisdom to ultimately make good decisions for themselves, and the professionals are seen as people who have the specialized knowledge to help illuminate the possibilities for them. Counseling must always increase possibilities. The professional, by listening and valuing the client, bolsters the client's confidence so that good decisions ultimately are made. For me, counseling is a mutually educative process that allows for the exchange of both information and affect. The aim of counseling is to help the client become better able to contend successfully with the specific problem at hand. Counseling as practiced by speech pathologists and audiologists should be problem centered with individuals who are emotionally upset by the problem at hand. This is opposed to psychotherapy, the province of specially trained professionals who are dealing with people who have chronic life adjustment problems. Many of the skills needed by both counselors and psychotherapists overlap considerably. It is the nature of the client and the nature of the problem that differ.

For us as speech and hearing professionals to be successful in counseling, we must help clients to become more *congruent*. A person's ability to function effectively in the world is a combination of the intellectual abilities (cognition) by which we process data and the emotions (affect) by which we intuit the world. When one is congruent, one has equal access to intellect and to affect, and decision making becomes easier because of an increased awareness of who and what one is. One is able to respond to a situation with both intellect and emotion; the behavior then is always self-enhancing. Total congruence is an idealized state that for most of us is achieved only at very special peak moments in life, but we as professionals need to be always striving to become more congruent in our lives, and we need to be working to always increase client congruence.

Most people tend to have their own particular style of internal organization. Some people are high in intellect and short on affect, and others are inclined to approach the world and personal problems from a feeling orientation with little recourse to information. Invariably these opposites are attracted to each other as they seek to achieve congruence via relationship, if not in the world. This is important for us to note when we are counseling couples; invariably they will be approaching the situation from different perspectives. The stress of a crisis, which often occurs around a communication disorder, tends to push people further into their cognitive or affective orientation. The cognitively oriented individuals want "just the facts," and the affect-oriented ones are so full of emotion that they cannot deal with any facts, presenting unique problems for the counselor.

For us to be effective at counseling, we must allow the affect-oriented person to ventilate feelings so that he or she then can begin to process the information that is needed, and we must help the intellectually oriented person gain access to feelings so as to become more congruent. This listening, valuing approach to counseling mandates that the speech and hearing professional be comfortable with the clients' feelings and develop skills to elicit them. I have found that this approach to counseling is very often frightening to many in our field. If we are not informing and we are not persuading, who are we? Gregory (1983) described the problem well when he commented about counseling stutterers:

> It may be that giving information expresses dominance and giving direction is related to manipulation and control. Whereas we may view listening and attempting to understand as being indecisive and uncertain. For whatever reason many student clinicians and professional speech–language pathologists seem to find it easier to be a provider of information and direction. (p. 10)

The notion of allowing and eliciting feelings is also frightening because of our mistaken notion that clients are emotionally fragile and somehow we can hurt them by allowing them to talk about and display their feelings. If one thinks about it, how can we hurt people by listening to them and valuing them? E. Webster (1977) said it well when she wrote:

> If counseling means the imposition of prescriptions without care for the person for whom they are prescribed, one may indeed do damage. The non-accepting, non-compassionate clinician runs the risk of hurting parents, so does the one who focuses concern on the child to the exclusion of concern for the parents. The speech pathologist or audiologist who leaves to others the interpretation of the information his field has to offer may do parents great harm. The same can be said for the clinician with limited knowledge who gives faulty information.
>
> On the other hand, it is virtually impossible for one person to damage another by listening to him, by trying to understand what the world looks like to him, by permitting him to express what is in him, and by honestly giving him the information he needs. In this view of counseling, the clinician serves as an accepting listener. He delays his judgement and tries to accept parents as they are and as they will become. (p. 337)

This text is, I hope, designed to help the speech and hearing professional expand to include other possibilities for relating to clients beyond informing and persuading. With that in mind, we need first to examine theory and how that theory has implications for our field; then we can look at the applications of a listening and valuing orientation to counseling clients.

2

Contemporary Theories of Counseling

There is an Indian parable about blind men and an elephant. Each man held on to a piece of the elephant and, when asked to describe the beast, each gave a very different version of the animal. Thus, the blind man who clutched the tail described the elephant as small, thin, and snakelike. The man clutching the leg described the elephant as very large and solid, whereas the one who had the trunk thought an elephant was flexible and strong. The point of the parable is that a person's view of reality depends on which part he or she is grasping and that perhaps every one of us has a limited view of reality at any given time.

A clinician trying to help a client manage change is much like one of the blind men in the parable. Clinicians operate from a theoretical framework that gives them a particular view of the "elephant." In practice, I think successful clinicians are eclectic in that they can and do mix their views, and are always evaluating which particular view is most useful in facilitating a therapeutic goal that fits the client context. Most counselors, however, still operate from a central tendency, that is, their theory of the therapeutic process, which serves as the organizing principles by which they tend to see client behavior.

With that in mind, let us examine the possible applications to four contemporary theories of counseling to the field of communication disorders: the behavioral, humanistic, existentialist, and cognitive models of counseling.

Behavioral Counseling

The behavioral model of counseling originated in the work of John Watson, with roots going back to Pavlov and his classically conditioned responses of a dog. Behaviorists concentrated on the strictly observable, with emphasis on external, environmental influences. (This emphasis was in sharp contrast to the subjectivity of the Freudian movement, which was beginning to invade American psychology around 1950, after many Freudians immigrated to the United States to avoid the Holocaust during World War II.) The leading proponent of behaviorism in the U.S. was B. F. Skinner. His seminal work, *Science and Human Behavior* (1953) became the basis of the clinical application of behaviorist notions to the alteration of maladaptive human behavior. Prior to that time, behaviorism was pretty much confined to academic laboratory exploration using experimental animals (mainly mice and pigeons) (Rimm & Cunningham, 1985).

Skinner contended that human behavior is shaped by the environment that "operates" on it: If a particular behavior is rewarded—that is, reinforced by the environment—that behavior will be repeated. Reinforcement is either positive, as when a reward is given when the desired behavior is elicited, or negative, as when an aversive stimulus is removed as a consequence of the individual's behavior. (Negative reinforcement is not to be confused with punishment, in which an aversive stimulus such as an electric shock is applied as a consequence of behavior.) The reinforcement, whether positive or negative, must be applied according to a precise schedule. The timing must be exact so that the person associates the reinforcement with the behavior (this does not have to be conscious, as we shall see briefly), and the reinforcer must be either desirable to the individual or aversive enough to cause the behavior to change. Strict behavioral psychologists believe that there is no freedom or choice: All behavior, they believe, is a product of external reinforcements.

The behavioral therapist designs therapy based on the observable. This is basically an "engineering" model of facilitating change in that a goal is set and the task is broken down into a series of small steps. Each successive approximation is achieved by the judicious application of reinforcement. As long as the reinforcer is appropriate, the timing of its application is precise, and the desired behavior is within the physiological capabilities of the organism (e.g., one cannot get an elephant to fly, Dumbo notwithstanding), then the behavior will change.

The story is told, perhaps apocryphally, of a psychology professor who was lecturing his class on operant conditioning techniques. The class decided, on its own, to condition the professor. Every time he moved to the right, the class would sit up, take notes, and appear to be interested (powerful reinforcers to any professor). As soon as he moved to the left, they would slump in their seats and appear to be quite inattentive. It was not long before he was lecturing from the doorway situated at the far right of the room. When the class got bored with this, they modified his behavior by reinforcing any movement to the left and pretty soon he was lecturing from the window. The professor, sophisticated as he was, responded much like any pigeon or mouse in a Skinner box, the apparent victim of the reinforcement schedule maintained by the class.

The fact that the behavior of humans can be changed as a result of the systematic application of reinforcement can be demonstrated both in laboratory conditions and in actual living conditions, and this approach has diverse applications to the field of speech pathology and audiology.

Application of Behaviorism to Communication Disorders

Behaviorism is a very attractive way of dealing with the deviant behaviors one encounters in a speech and hearing clinic. It provides a structured framework by which the therapist (especially the beginning therapist) can specify the particular behavior to be changed and, by breaking down the task into a series of successive approximations, can modify the deviant behavior. Progress at each stage can be measured. Perkins (1977) commented,

> Because speech therapy is just as behavioral as behavior modification (the former derived pragmatically, the latter from operant learning principles), the same general therapeutic considerations underlie most of the methods for remediating speech. . . . In a word, the clinician must begin where his client can perform without failure and by careful selection of types and schedules of reinforcement, move step by step to the terminal goal. No step is taken until its success is assured. At the first sign of failure, the therapist mounts a strategic retreat to a point at which successful performance can be established. (p. 379)

Behavior modification techniques have been and still are used quite extensively in our field. The principles of behavior modification are relatively easy to teach to students, and the structure of the approach allays a great deal of therapeutic anxiety. The concrete nature of many of the techniques can be quite seductive to novice therapists. The 1970s, when behavior modification took hold in our field, seemed to be what could be called the "Fruit Loop" decade. One could rarely stick one's head into a therapy observation room without seeing a student clinician reinforcing a child's behavior with a Fruit Loop.

The literature is replete with behavior modification schemes. To name a few, Shames and Florance (1982) recommended a behavioral approach to shaping fluency in young stutterers; Moore (1982) recommended behavioral modification to eliminate or reduce vocal abuse; Cottrel, Montague, Farb, and Throne (1980) utilized operant techniques for teaching vocabulary to developmentally delayed children. Operant techniques have been used extensively in audiology to condition difficult-to-test populations to respond to sound (Lloyd, Spradlin, & Reid, 1968; Yarnell, 1983).

Among the many studies using the operant approach, two stand out. The study of Stech, Curtiss, Troesch, and Binnie (1973) described the ways in which the client conditions and shapes the therapist's behavior. (The client strikes back!) Perhaps the ultimate study in behaviorism in our field is Starkweather's (1974) scheme to condition the student clinician, via earphones, while the student was conditioning the client. (One wonders who was conditioning the supervisor.)

Limitations of Behaviorism

The behavioral approach presupposes a very narrow view of the speech and hearing clinician's role and responsibilities, reducing the clinical task to one of dispensing Fruit Loops. The mystery and art of client–clinician relationships are not developed. This approach also leaves unattended the issue of carryover into the client's environment. Behaviorism would predict that a number of reinforcers in the client's environment are maintaining the deviant behavior, and these reinforcers are not addressed by working solely with the client. The behavioral approach is clearly able to modify superficial behavior but does not deal with such nebulous concepts as personal growth, self-esteem, and anxiety because it is hard to specify the overt behaviors of these phenomena; however, these concepts may have considerable effect on communication behavior and may be very useful for accomplishing therapeutic change.

A consequence of the unrealistic use of behaviorism to control behavior may be the loss of altruism. Philosophers and psychologists have postulated that humans are one species that demonstrates altruistic behavior: that is, doing good for the sake of doing good. (Although a strict behaviorist might say we do good because it feels good and thus we get reinforced for altruistic behavior.) Nevertheless, I think behaviorism would encourage a "What's in it for me attitude," which in turn would encourage superficial changes in behavior to conform to the extrinsic reinforcer. It remains to be seen whether a child, for example, can see good speech as something valuable in its own right or as a tedious prerequisite to getting a reward; if it is the latter, there is little likelihood of carryover outside of the therapy room.

It is also clear that we do have choices about our behavior (a notion that behaviorists resist). If the college professor who was conditioned by the class had been made aware of what was happening, he could have resisted the conditioning and lectured from the center of the room, albeit discomforted by the fact that the class appeared to be asleep. It is our awareness of what is happening to us and our willingness to assume responsibility for how we behave that will enable us to control environmental reinforcers; the reinforcers may not be as powerful in shaping behavior in humans as they appear to be in laboratory animals.

Humanistic Counseling

Parallel with the development of behaviorism in the United States was the development of humanistic psychology, known as the "third force" in American psychology (i.e., third after Freudian psychoanalysis and Watsonian behaviorism). The theoretical and clinical underpinnings of the humanistic movement in the United States were provided by Carl Rogers and Abraham Maslow. Maslow (1962) postulated that humans have an innate drive to grow—he termed this drive *self-actualization*. The self-actualization drive is very frequently thwarted by teaching and parenting that direct the child to look to others for approval and wisdom. The goal of therapy is to help the person remove the barriers to the self-actualizing drive and learn to respond to the realm of inner promptings, where true wisdom lies.

A book written by psychiatrist Sheldon Kopp gives an excellent description of the humanistic therapeutic process. The book has the marvelous title of *If you Meet the Buddha on the Road Kill Him!* (1972), which comes from an old Buddhist admonition that any Buddha one meets on the road must be a false one, since the true Buddha is within oneself. As you can see, the roots of humanism are quite ancient. Lao-tze, a Chinese sage who wrote 2,500 years ago, articulated the humanistic credo so well when he wrote,

> If I keep from meddling with people, they take care of themselves.
> If I keep from commanding people, they behave themselves.
> If I keep from preaching at people, they improve themselves.
> If I keep from imposing on people, they become themselves.
> (cited in Bynner, 1962, p. 32)

The application of humanistic principles to the clinical population is reflected in the monumental works of Carl Rogers. His seminal work, *Client Centered Therapy* (1951), marked an ideological turning point in contemporary clinical psychology (Arbuckle, 1970). At that time, psychologists were concerned mainly with vocational counseling, intelligence testing, and personality evaluations. The client-centered counseling of Rogers placed little emphasis on diagnosis and testing; it stressed the quality of the interpersonal relationship as the means for promoting client growth. According to Rogers, there are three preconditions for change within a therapeutic environment. First, the counselor must develop an unconditional regard for the client so that the client feels free to express anything he or she wants to. This is fostered by nonjudgmental listening and valuing of the client within a relationship that promotes total acceptance. The client is never given a label such as "neurotic," or "mentally retarded," but is always accepted on his or her own terms.

Second, the counselor must practice empathetic listening, what Rogers refers to as hearing the "faint knocking." This is sometimes referred to as reflective listening and is the most seemingly teachable of humanistic techniques. Unfortunately, if the technique is practiced without empathy, it will fail miserably, as it usually does in the hands of a novice practitioner who is focused on techniques and not on the client. (This is discussed further in Chapter 6.) In empathetic listening, the counselor reflects back to the client the feelings conveyed in the message.

The third condition, and probably the most difficult to achieve, is that of counselor congruence. Rogers (1980) wrote,

> When my experiencing of this moment is present in my awareness and when what is present in my awareness is present in my communication, then each of these three levels matches or is congruent. At such moments I am integrated or whole, I am completely in one piece. Most of the time, I, like everyone else, exhibit some degree of incongruence. I have learned, however, that realness, or genuineness, or congruence—whatever term you wish to give it—is a fundamental basis for the best of communication. (p. 15)

Counselor congruence demands that the counselor be in touch with his or her own needs and experiences. It suggests a wholeness for the counselor to be "there" completely for the client. Armed then with an unconditional regard, empathy, and congruence, the counselor enters into a therapeutic alliance with the client so as to release the client's self-actualizing drive. Client-centered therapy assumes that with these facilitative conditions, the client's vast resources for self-understanding and growth will be tapped and change will occur.

Application of Humanism to Communication Disorders

Speech pathology and audiology have a long humanistic history, going back to some of our earliest practitioners. Backus and Beasley (1951) felt that "speech therapy more and more is shifting away from an orientation based primarily upon devices, toward one based primarily on therapeutic relationships" (p. 2).

Cooper (1966) reported that for stutterers, client progress was related to the nature of the affect interchange between the client and the clinician. He also noted that important similarities exist between stuttering therapy and psychotherapy. E. Webster (1966, 1977) consistently argued for a humanistic counseling model for the speech pathologist/audiologist especially in relationship to parents, but also in therapeutic encounters. Caracciolo, Rigrodsky, and Morrison (1978) reported on the use of a Rogerian nondirective approach in the supervision of student clinicians. Their hope was that if the supervisor modeled the Rogerian approach to the student clinician, the would-be clinician could transfer this to the client relationship. Currently in the field of communication disorders, probably no one has been as consistently humanistic in both clinical behavior and writing as Albert Murphy (1982), who wrote,

> Happiness in the noblest sense comes in large measure through helping relationships with others, stretching our professional resources and the resource of the mind and the heart. Every now and then something in our deeper selves enables us to realize that what truly counts in life is not a matter of what is in you or what is in me but of what occurs between us. That divine spark of relationship may be the most fundamental life force of all. (p. 473)

Limitations of the Humanistic Model

The problem with the humanistic approach is how to apply it to the field of communication disorders. The concepts of congruence, empathy, and self-actualization are nebulous and are not readily amenable to measurement or, for that matter, to the teaching and training of student clinicians. Humanism requires a leap of faith: With the right therapeutic environment, the self-actualizing drive will bubble through. Thus, clinicians are left in a potentially uncomfortable, unstructured framework. Humanism demands that the clinician yield power to the client to determine the course of therapy—the "lesson plan" is thrown out or, better, is devised by both the client and the clinician in a spontaneous, egalitarian manner. Humanism places a great deal of responsibility on the client and demands a great deal of self-confidence on the part of the clinician.

Clinicians must learn behavior that appears to be contrary to what is usually thought of as professional. They must listen instead of prescribe. A humanistic approach is very difficult, especially for a young, insecure therapist who doesn't have the experience and confidence necessary to allow for an unstructured, spontaneous interchange with the client. It is also difficult to see how to apply the humanistic precepts to difficult clinical populations such as children and adults with severe brain damage, as well as to very young children in general.

Counseling and Existentialism

Paralleling the development of humanism in the United States was the growth of existential philosophy in Europe. The existentialists emerged upon the rediscovery by the French intellectual movement of the work of the mid-nineteenth century Danish philosopher Kierkegaard (Yalom, 1980). Existential philosophers were attempting to look at the problems of human existence without the comfort provided by traditional religious thought. To the existentialists, the problems of living are related to the facts of existence, namely, that we must die, that we have freedom, that we are alone, and that life is meaningless.

Existential notions also became the basis of an approach to psychotherapy. Therapists such as Frankl, Fromm, and May began to use existential philosophy as a basis for understanding and examining the problems presented by their patients. Almost all of the existential therapists were latter-day psychoanalysts. In traditional psychoanalytic thought, anxiety is seen as the motivating force for a patient's deviant behavior. The source of the anxiety for the traditional Freudian is the conflict between the instinctual drives such as Thanatos (death) and Eros (life) or between the id (the pleasure drive) and the superego (the social restrictions as incorporated within the infant by the parent in the form of the conscience). The resultant anxiety from these conflicts is the source of neurotic behavior.

Existential psychotherapy is a dynamic therapy that also postulates anxiety as the motivating force. For the existential psychotherapist, however, anxiety occurs when the individual confronts the facts of existence: death, freedom (which involves responsibility), loneliness, and meaninglessness. Neurotic behavior for the existential psychologists arises from the avoidance of dealing with the basic issues of existence. Existentialists do not take a developmental view of behavior in that they are not especially concerned with promoting insight into people's early history in order to understand current behavior. This is contrasted with traditional psychotherapy, which is historically based and seeks to help patients gain insight into their past in order to understand their present behavior.

Existentialism is a very "here and now" therapy that focuses on the present and sees the client's current behavior as reflecting some clash with one of the existential issues. The avoidance of the existential issues is viewed as creating the anxiety that ultimately gets us into interpersonal or intrapersonal difficulties. Let us look at each of the existential issues.

Death

Death, the single most important issue of life, is a topic that most people avoid. Mitford (1963) pointed out how funeral directors increase their profits by catering to our death avoidance, providing elegant clothing for the deceased, a soft and buoyant mattress, and of course the marvelous euphemism of a "slumber room" for the last viewing of the elegant coffin that contains the "sleeping" corpse. The existential philosophers tell us that if we continue with death avoidance, we will live a life with death anxiety—one in which we tend to postpone things and procrastinate without fully appreciating our everyday existence. If we do not recognize the boundaries of our existence, we tend to avoid enjoying the commonplace. (After all, we are going to live forever!) The fear of death is always greatest in those who feel that they have not lived their lives fully. According to Yalom (1989), "A good working formula is the more unlived the life or unrealized potential, the greater the death anxiety" (p. 6).

On the other hand, with death awareness, persons savor and enjoy every moment of the day. They are aware of how transitory and finite life is; they do not squander their time.

Yalom (1980) found the following changes in the lives of cancer patients as they came to grips with their impending death:

A rearrangement of life's priorities; a trivializing of the trivial.

A sense of liberation, being able to choose not to do those things that they do not wish to do.

An enhanced sense of living in the immediate present rather than postponing life until retirement or some other part of the future.

A vivid appreciation of the elemental facts of life, the changing seasons, the wind, falling leaves, the last Christmas.

Deeper communication with loved ones than before the crisis.

Fewer interpersonal fears, less concerns about rejection, greater willingness to take risks than before the crisis. (p. 64)

We are all terminal. How nice it would be if we could all develop death awareness without having cancer. Unfortunately, for most people, living with death awareness comes about only as a result of a life crisis.

Responsibility

The existentialists are unyielding on the issue of responsibility. It is the basis of their therapy. To an existential therapist/philosopher, each person is responsible for his or her life and for constituting his or her reality.

Existence is you doing you! This uncompromising position leaves an individual feeling very uncomfortable because there is no one else to blame for failure. For an existentialist, an individual is making choices at all times, including the choice of how to respond to an event in life. For example, although a person does not choose to be born deaf or to have a stroke, the person does have a choice about how to deal with it. David Wright (1969), a poet and a deafened adult, has written elegantly about his deafness and about disabilities in general. He found many positives:

> The handicapped are less at the mercy of vague unhappiness that afflicts so many, especially those without aim in life, whose consequent boredom promotes what used to be called spleen. The disabled have been given a built-in, ready-packed objective which is always present; a definite impediment to get the better of. Like the prospect of hanging, it concentrates the faculties wonderfully. (p. 111)

As a counselor, one never feels sorry for a client, because the client always has a choice about what to do about the disorder; the responsibility of choice also allows an opportunity to grow. I think responsibility assumption is the basis of all change and growth. The first step in all therapeutic changes is responsibility assumption. If one feels no responsibility for one's predicament, then how can one change it?

The pathology of responsibility evasion can range from the profound to the commonplace, and in some way, we all try more or less to evade responsibility. Erich Fromm (1941), in his classic book *Escape from Freedom,* asserted that, on a societal level, freedom engenders anxiety; hence, totalitarian forms of government developed as a protection against the responsibility required to maintain a democracy. There is probably no more common occurrence of responsibility evasion than in the addicted personality of the smoker or the alcoholic. Smoking or drinking is not something that happens to a person; it is something a person does to himself or herself. The smoker or the alcoholic may feel as if he or she *has to* smoke a cigarette or have a drink, but the existential truth of the matter is that the person is choosing to smoke or drink. (There is evidence that alcoholics, in particular, have a different physiological response to alcohol than nonalcoholics, but this must never be an excuse; it still comes down to choice.)

Addicts who are going to succeed in quitting are the ones who assume responsibility for their own behavior, recognizing that nobody is going to make the change for them. They also need a great deal of emotional support, such as that provided by groups like Alcoholics Anonymous. It is never easy to give up an addiction, but without responsibility assumption, it is impossible. The existentialists are unyielding on responsibility assumption. One cannot even complain about the weather! I like the Ralph Waldo Emerson quote that "This would be a perfect day if we but knew what to do with it!" So, even with "bad" weather, it is our responsibility to make a good day of it.

Loneliness

Each of us is alone in the universe; after birth, we can no longer merge with anyone else. According to existentialists, almost all anxiety of childhood stems from the awareness of separation. The infant, who is not capable of surviving on his or her own, cannot bear to be separated from the parents because separation is death. Thus is born people's terror of separation and loneliness. Yet we are alone, and that crushing fact is central to existential thought. When we experience existential loneliness, we find our mature love.

Anxiety of loneliness gives rise to romantic love, the kind that is described in song lyrics, the kind that states, "I will die if you leave me." Romantic love fosters a mutually dependent relationship in which there is no growth. Scott Peck (1978), who devoted a considerable portion of his book *The Road Less Traveled* to a discussion of love, sees romantic love as a biological "trap" planned by nature to ensure marriage and the survival of the species. Romantic love may also be an evolutionary step on the way to mature love, which Peck defines as "the will to extend one's self for the purpose of nurturing one's own or another's spiritual growth" (p. 81). All definitions of mature love involve a separation that allows for growth.

The route to mature love may be through a crisis experience that brings us face to face with our existential loneliness. Moustakes (1961), who has written extensively about the loneliness experience and how it relates to love, recounted his experience when he had to make a decision regarding major surgery for his critically ill daughter:

> It was a terrible responsibility, being required to make a life or death decision, for someone else. This awful feeling, this overwhelming sense of responsibility, I could not share with anyone. I felt utterly alone, entirely lost and frightened; my existence was absorbed in the crisis. No one fully understood my terror or how this terror gave impetus to deep feelings of loneliness and isolation which had been dormant within me. There at the center of my being, loneliness aroused me to a self-awareness I had never known before. (p. 2)

Encountering our loneliness is a means of finding our unconditional regard for humanity. It is a "boundary experience," much like death awareness, which promotes self-growth. The love that stems from our loneliness encounter can be a love that comes from the richness of ourselves. In the giving of it we renew ourselves.

Meaninglessness

For the existentialists, there is no extrinsic meaning to the world. For them, we are huddled on this planet hurtling through space in the face of cosmic indifference. The meaninglessness of the universe is central to existential thought in that the discovery of meaning for human beings is that which they construct for themselves. There is no "objective" truth, only a subjective one that is, therefore, highly individualistic. There is a world out there, but it is given form and substance only by human interpretation. In the face of a meaningless world, we must construct our own vision of the purpose and meaning in life. Thus, one could take a traditional religious view (e.g., "We are here to fulfill God's design"), an altruistic view (e.g., "We are here to do good"), a dedicated view (e.g., "We are here to solve a particular problem"), a humanistic view (e.g., "We are here to self-actualize"), or a hedonistic view (e.g., "We are here to have a good time").

An existential therapist is always seeking to understand the client's particular view of the world. For existential therapists, there is never any judgment of good or bad; it is a matter of understanding what is, and proceeding from there.

Application of Existentialism to Communication Disorders

Existential thought has a very wide application to our field. The existential issues abound within all our clinical interactions. Since I have discovered the vocabulary and notions of the existentialists, I feel the excitement of the Molière character who discovers that he has been speaking prose all his life. Yalom (1980) commented that psychiatrists do not deal with these issues because they have not resolved them for themselves. I think that statement is partly true for me, but I have also needed the theoretical framework in order to see client behavior and to work through for myself many of these issues. Farran, Keane-Hagerty, Salloway, Kupferer, and Wilkin (1991) found the existential issues abounding in the caregivers of Alzheimer's patients. It was through suffering that the caregivers were able to assume responsibility for themselves and find meaning in their lives. My wife's illness has also helped us to live authentically, making everything count, and has given meaning and focus to our life.

The death issue is always present in our clinical work. In many cases, we are dealing with people who have undergone a traumatic change. All change involves a death in that we must give up and lose something. (We also get something, but we don't always recognize it at the time.) Parents of deaf children must give up the dream of having a normal child and also of their having a "normal" life. The aphasic client and his or her family may have to give up the person as a viable communicating human being; this is a death. Many of our clients have literally had near-death experiences, especially those undergoing laryngectomies or strokes. This can leave them very frightened as they realize their vulnerability, or mobilized as they realize how little time they have left. M. Webster (1982), a speech pathologist who suffered a stroke, found that with recovery "things like trees, flowers, sunsets and friends and loved ones are more appreciated" (p. 237).

Death awareness mobilizes the client and the clinician. When you are aware that death can touch you at any time, you abandon timidity; you want to extract the most from every encounter and you recognize that nothing is permanent. For the clinician, termination is an important clinical tool. All meetings need to have a very definite closure. Group meetings become more intense as the hour for termination draws near. Clients are motivated to work hard when they know that they have a very limited time to be with the clinician. There is experimental support for these notions. Shlien, Mosak, and Dreikors (1962) found that patients within a time-limited counseling program made more progress than did patients within a counseling program with no imposed time limits. Munro and Bach (1975) found that college students seeking counseling services showed significantly more gains in self-acceptance and increased independence when they were enrolled in time-limited therapy (eight sessions) than did a control group of students who had no time limitation.

When both clinician and client recognize that there is limited time, the emphasis in therapy becomes one of quality of endeavor. Time, per se, does not heal; only activity does. However, with an awareness of time limitation comes an increase in activity and an increase in risk.

The freedom/responsibility issue is vital to any therapeutic progress and to any carryover of the behavior into the client's life. In my own observations of many therapeutic relationships, I have often seen clinicians fail to give responsibility for choice and behavior to the client. I often find that there is so much "rescuing" that the clients are not empowered and therefore do not grow. Geri Jewell ("ASHA Interview," 1983), an actress with cerebral palsy, felt that the biggest impediment to her growing up was that teachers had low expectations for her and did not require her to assume responsibility. One sees the problem of low expectations repeatedly in the deaf population. White (1982) reported on a series of workshops he conducted with teachers and counselors at six schools for the deaf. Two hundred eighty-one participants were asked to rank 24 social competencies lacking among the deaf. The social issue ranked first by almost all participants was "taking responsibility for own actions."

Hornyak (1980), using the language of transactional analysis, pointed out the dangers for the speech pathologists in "rescuing" clients, which robs them of their autonomy and keeps them feeling powerless. In the therapy contact, according to Hornyak, the client should be perceived as a human being who is not helpless.

When professionals become the ultimate rescuers of the people they are helping, they limit growth and keep clients from assuming responsibility for their own behavior. Somehow we must teach the stutterers to take responsibility for their nonfluency, the dysphonics for their vocal behavior, and the articulatory defectives for their misarticulations. They must realize that the change comes from inside rather than from external sources. When clients recognize and experience their own powers and responsibilities, they can alter specific speech behavior and maintain changes outside the therapeutic relationship.

The loneliness notion has wide application to our field. To have a communication disorder is to be cut off from contact with others. This is very anxiety provoking. I experience this anxiety every time I am in the deaf community. My sign language skills are very limited, almost nonexistent, despite three beginning sign language courses in which I finally learned how to distinguish *D* from *F.* In the presence of people who are facile with sign language and for whom that is their primary means of communication, I am a severely handicapped individual. I am frightened, I hope people will not approach, and I seek to leave the situation at the first opportunity. After leaving a group of deaf people, I often think how it must be for them to deal with the hearing world on an everyday basis: One could only feel isolated and lonely, and eager to encounter someone with whom to communicate.

As a practicing audiologist, it became apparent to me that the underlying terror of progressive hearing loss experienced by some clients resulted from the feeling of being cut off and isolated. The major means by which we alleviate our interpersonal loneliness is verbal communication, and when that is difficult, we become disturbed. The child who would not let his mother out of sight because he could not hear her when she was in a different room in the house, the truck driver who burst into tears because he could not go to the bar with his cronies as he no longer heard the punch line of the jokes they told, and the wife complaining about her hearing-impaired husband who refused to go out of the house because communication was so difficult for him, are, in one form or another, loneliness experiences. The stutterer who limits his contact with people, the laryngectomized adult who refuses to leave his home, and the individual with a cleft palate who avoids contact with people because his speech and appearance are so poor are also very lonely.

Probably the loneliest of all is the adult with brain damage who is locked into his personal "cell" with blocked communication doors and windows. We must break through these doors; alleviating a communication disorder is an incredibly tender and beautiful thing to do. There are not many more important gifts that we can bring to others.

Any catastrophic change in a person's life becomes a loneliness experience because the person is cut off from all of the usual sources of support. Parents and friends seldom understand the person's pain of loss because they are so busy trying to make the person "feel better" that they do not respond to the grief; they also feel very awkward and don't know how to approach the individual who has experienced the tragedy.

Suzanne Massie, the mother of hemophiliac Bobby, wrote,

> The ostracism and isolation were almost harder to adapt to than the disease itself. More than ever we needed the help and comfort of close human contact. We needed friends. In our situation they were essential. I cannot remember a single friend who was near us in the early days of Bobby's illness. . . . It was as though we were living on an island. (Massie & Massie, 1973, p. 148)

The encounter with crisis, as Moustakes (1961) found with his child, in itself puts us in touch with our existential loneliness. How nice it would be to find a helping, empathetic friend at that time who just listens to us.

The existential issue of meaninglessness also emerges full blown from crises. All of us have a cosmological view—that is, a way of explaining to ourselves how things operate in the world. Most people would like to impose on the universe an order and a rationality that existentialists tell us really does not exist. We need to find a reason for the tragedy, some way to explain it. The most common explanation is that God in heaven punishes the wicked and rewards the good: When something bad befalls us, we feel that we must have been wicked. (This is why in many cultures children with disabilities are hidden, because they are believed to represent some "sin" that the parent committed.) The converse of this is that God is wicked, which poses a huge dilemma for most people undergoing a crisis in their lives; it involves a very painful reevaluation of their cosmological view. The deeply religious will often say, "This awful thing that has happened is part of God's grand design for me, but because I am only human I cannot perceive the total tapestry of God's intent."

Suzanne Massie, a deeply religious woman, had to wrestle with this big cosmic question of why:

> And yet the need to find meaning remains. . . . Why, God, why?
> I could not consider Bobby's hemophilia punishment. When I looked at my bright-eyed child, full of energy and drive, it was unthinkable that God would meaninglessly visit His wrath upon him. . . . Could it be to teach us suffering? The Russians saw in suffering a way to enlightenment. To them it was not a curse but a mystery with great potential for good. "Be glad Suzanne," Svetlana would say to me. "Be glad you feel deeply." "And remember," she would say, "You are a queen,

because you are suffering." In the Soviet Union, a friend told me with respect, "Hemophilia is your family struggle; through it you have been able to glimpse the suffering of our Lord."

In time I came to believe. In time I became grateful that we had been given the chance to see and feel so much. And I told Bobby this, that he had been given suffering earlier than many but that inevitably suffering and failure come to all in life. I told him he was fortunate to have had the chance to meet it when he was young, because those who meet it early are luckier than those whom it comes to later, when it often breaks them. (Massie & Massie, 1973, p. 148)

All of our cognizant clients are constantly struggling with the issue of meaning. Those who are less religious are left with a void that they somehow must fill. Successful families and successful clients, as we shall see later, are those who find some meaning in the tragedies that have befallen them. Therapists must be willing to help the clients find their own meaning to resolve the "why me" crisis. This often means participating in or listening to "God talk," an area that is very uncomfortable for most therapists.

The existential issues also have cogency for us as professionals; through death awareness we can restore our zest in our work, for clinicians who live with death awareness cannot be bored. Responsibility assumption leads to our personal and professional growth; through loneliness we can find the mature love that truly nurtures our clients, and the resolution of meaninglessness gives rise to our commitment.

Limitations of Existentialism

Existential therapy is much more a philosophy than a therapeutic technique, so there is very little for a clinician to grasp in working with clients; it demands that we stay with what we and the client know and can observe. Existentialists are very "now" oriented and are seeking to explain behavior in terms of the relevant existential issues, but there is no unifying strategy for evoking the issue. Clinicians are left to flounder on their own.

Use of existentialism in clinical interactions would exceed the traditional boundaries for most speech pathologists and audiologists. For example, we would find ourselves involved in a great deal of "God talk" with many of our clients. Existentialism demands of us as individuals and as professionals a maturity that we may not now possess, but it will possibly be the avenue for our future growth. For me, an awareness of existentialism keeps me focused and grounded in what is important in life.

Cognitive Therapy

The cognitive approach to therapy offers a fourth view of the therapeutic "elephant." The underlying concept of cognitive therapy is that emotional disorder is basically a disorder of thinking. The cognitive therapist helps clients to identify the specific misconceptions and unrealistic expectations in their thinking that underlie their behavior, and then forces clients to test the validity of their assumptions against reality. It is a highly confrontational approach in that the client is always challenged to examine the underlying "irrational" assumptions that are reflected in his or her language and behavior. A cognitive therapist is not concerned with the person's past history, but is concerned only with the meaning that the client attributes to an event. A cognitive therapist is not directly interested in the emotions—the underlying assumption is that "as you think is how you feel" and if we straighten out your thinking, we will straighten out your feelings. Of the many cognitive therapists, the leading proponent was Albert Ellis, the founder of rational–emotive therapy. He developed a list of the irrational ideas that most of his clients presented to him in one form or another. The following irrational ideas are adapted from his text (Ellis, 1977).

- It is a dire necessity for an adult human to be loved or approved of by virtually every "significant other" in his or her community.

- A person should be thoroughly competent, adequate, and achieving in all possible respects if he or she is to consider himself or herself worthwhile, and he or she is utterly worthless if he is incompetent in any way.

- Certain people can be labeled bad, wicked, or villainous, and they deserve severe blame or punishment for their sins.

- It is awful or catastrophic when things are not the way an individual would very much like them to be.

- Human unhappiness is externally caused, and individuals have little or no ability to control their sorrows and disturbances.

- If something is or may be dangerous or fearsome, one should be terribly concerned about it and should keep dwelling on the possibility of its occurrence.

- It is easier to avoid certain life difficulties and self-responsibilities than it is to face them.

- An individual should be dependent on others and needs someone stronger than himself or herself on whom to rely.

- A person's past history is an all-important determinant of his or her present behavior, and because something once strongly affected his or her life, it should continue to do so.

- An individual should become quite upset over other people's problems and disturbances.

- There is invariably a correct, precise, and perfect solution to human problems, and it is catastrophic if this perfect solution is not found.

Applications to Communication Disorders

I think cognitive therapy is a model of counseling that is used a great deal in our field without our recognizing it as such. We use this approach when we set about to persuade clients, as when we list the reasons why someone should get a hearing aid or use an artificial larynx. We are not concerned with the client's feelings, assuming that once the person gets the appliance and sees how well it functions, the feelings will change.

A more systematic application of cognitive therapy has been with fluency disorders. Maxwell (1982) reported that a majority of his clients showed a significant reduction in the severity of their stuttering and a marked decline in speech-related stress under a therapeutic regime that employed various self-management and self-monitoring strategies. Emerick (1988) outlined in detail a cognitive approach to be used with adult stutterers.

I find Ellis's (1977) ideas immensely useful in almost all of my professional and personal contacts. Irrational ideas are reflected in the language people use to describe their problems; for example, the use of the word *can't* when it is really a "choose not to" situation, as in, "I can't tell my pediatrician how angry I am," or, "I can't use my new speech on the telephone." Translation: "I choose not to." Other language changes that I find valuable are as follows:

- "Should" and "ought" changed to "want to" or "not want to," as in, "I should use my new voice" to "I want to (or do not want to) use my new voice."

- "Have to" changed to "want to" or "choose to," as in, "I have to stay home and not meet people," to, "I want to stay home," or, "I choose to stay home."

- "We," "us," "society," and so on, changed to "I," as in "We are unhappy with this class," to, "I am unhappy with this class (therefore I can do something about it if I choose to)."

- Modified "to be" verbs, as in, "I am a dumb person," to, "I did a dumb thing and I am still a smart person."

- "But" changed to "and" (as in all the "yes . . . but" sentences), as in, "I want to speak in public but I am afraid," to, "I want to speak in public and I am afraid."

All of these linguistic changes force the person to assume responsibility for his or her behavior and for thinking clearly about that behavior. Underlying rational–emotive therapy, as with all other therapies, is responsibility assumption. I find that when I listen for the irrational assumptions that are reflected in the language of the client, and when I gently change the language, there is often immense benefit to the client.

I find that irrational ideas such as, "I must be universally liked," and "A competent and worthwhile person makes no mistakes" are particularly valuable in working with student clinicians, as well as with professionals. These people generally try so hard to be liked that they are unwilling to offend their clients in any way. Thus, students and clinicians tend to meet client expectations rather than their own. The fear of making mistakes severely limits personal and professional growth and seems to be almost epidemic in student populations. I think that this is a direct reflection of the poor teaching methods that our students have been subjected to—teaching that does not accept mistakes and incompetency as natural to the learning process. Almost every professional group with which I work is beset by these same issues, and professional growth is usually limited by the unwillingness to assume risk.

Limitations of Cognitive Counseling

The rational–emotive therapies were developed for neurotic individuals whose emotions were irrational or, more accurately, whose feelings were in significant disparity with objective reality. The clients we are dealing with in communication disorders have very strong emotions, as we shall see in Chapter 4, and these feelings are based on a reality. It is very normal, very appropriate, and very rational to feel bad because you have a deaf child, an aphasic husband, or a severe hearing loss. My own personal bias is that these feelings need expression and need to be acknowledged in order for counseling to move forward. A strictly cognitive approach cuts short the expression of feelings and moves clients quickly (I think too quickly) into the intellectual realm.

The other limitation of the cognitive therapies is the ever-present likelihood of getting into a persuasion model of counseling. A very fine line exists between cognitive restructuring and persuading. Counselors need to point out "irrationality" without prescribing. It is very difficult to do this. By prescribing, one may help to create the dependent client who does not think for himself or herself—the reverse of what any good counselor would want. The temptation to get the client to think as we do is very great, but this must be avoided if we are to be truly helpful. When we set out to persuade, we stop listening. We are so busy marshaling our arguments that we do not hear what the client is really saying, and this can be detrimental to client growth.

The Theories Compared

These, then, are four views of the therapeutic "elephant" that I think have much relevance for our field. In theory, the approaches are very divergent; in practice, there are many more similarities than differences. To contrast them, we can use an example of a man going to a counselor to try to give up smoking. A behavioral therapist would devise a plan of cigarette reduction and periodic rewards for meeting the reduction criterion. A client-centered therapist would begin by asking the client what he thought needed to be done in order to give up smoking, and together they might devise a plan. The existential therapist would point out to the client that smoking is something he is choosing to do and perhaps he is now ready to choose something else. The cognitive therapist would direct the client to examine the irrational assumption he is making, namely, that lung cancer and all of the other known negative effects of smoking cannot happen to him.

In practice, latter-day behaviorists recognize fully the importance of the therapeutic relationship in promoting growth. Behavioral therapists have come to recognize that one of the first goals of the counselor is to establish a relationship with clients in which the clients feel free to express themselves to the counselors and in which the counselor is perceived as someone who is interested in attempting to help with the problem. It is also the clients who select the goals of therapy and, in concert with the therapist, work to change the environmental reinforcers that are maintaining the current self-defeating behaviors (Hansen, Stavis, & Warner, 1977). This view of counseling could be written by any humanist-oriented counselor. By the same token, Yalom (1975) (no behaviorist, he) commented that "every form of psychotherapy is a learning process relying in part on operant conditioning" (p. 57). Cognitive therapists and existentialists would agree wholeheartedly on the issue of meaning, and humanists are very much allied with existentialists, although they tend to be a bit more upbeat and less philosophically based then their existential counterparts. All therapists agree that no change can take place without responsibility assumption by the client. The particular routes to that goal vary, but many of the therapeutic roads cross one another.

No experimental evidence supports the superiority of any one of these counseling approaches. The variables that need to be controlled in order to determine scientifically which is a better approach (e.g., counselor competency, purity of counselor theory, level of client maladjustment, and degree of and measurement of change) are currently so intangible as to preclude any meaningful research into therapeutic efficacy. We are reduced to selecting a particular approach because it is most congenial to our personality and to our worldview. The client behavior exists, and it is a matter of which therapeutic lens the counselor selects in order to see it.

The general theory that an individual holds about counseling is a reflection of his or her attitudes about humans and how they learn, change, and grow. Theory in this context becomes synonymous with "point of view," which, in turn, reflects how the counselor views client behavior. The problem with theory is that it can quickly become dogma and thus severely limit the response of the counselor. I think that we must choose a particular way of approaching clients and then be willing to adapt within the context of the client–clinician relationship. My own personal view, which will be expounded later, is that all good counseling begins from careful listening and that the client will teach us how to be most helpful.

3

Erikson Life Cycle and Relationship

Among the pantheon of my personal gurus, Erik Erikson rates highly. The son of a Jewish mother, a Christian father, and a Jewish stepfather, he came of age in Germany during the rise of Hitler. As a youth he was an itinerant artist, a euphemism for a young man without much direction. He was employed as a tutor in a family that was friendly with Freud. Anna Freud, trained as an elementary school teacher, was interested in applying psychoanalytic therapy—developed by her father—to the raising of children, and became involved with the family that Erikson was tutoring. Erikson was swept up in the psychoanalytic movement and entered psychoanalysis (which was a requirement for anyone seeking to become a psychoanalyst) with Anna Freud. He finished his psychoanalytic training in 1933 and, because of the deteriorating conditions in Germany and his Jewish family connections, emigrated with his family to the United States. He worked in Boston for several years as a child analyst, one of the first analysts in the United States to specialize in children.

Erikson subsequently moved to the west coast, studied the child-raising practices of the Sioux and Yurok tribes, and worked with the children enrolled at the Institute of Child Welfare in California. He became quite interested in how culture shapes personality and, with the eye of a painter and the training of a clinician, he observed the evolution of the life cycle from infancy to death. Among Erikson's many works, probably the most outstanding is his *Childhood and Society* (1950), in which he first delineated his observation of the life cycle. (Readers interested in further investigating the life and work of Erikson are referred to the excellent biography written by Robert Coles, 1970.)

Erikson's frequently used and quoted model of the life cycle is an immensely useful way to look at the developing ego qualities that emerge during critical periods of development from childhood to adulthood. Erikson felt that each successive stage has a special relationship to a basic element of society because the life cycle and our institutions have evolved together. Each stage of ego development or "crisis" needs to be resolved, at least partially, before one can successfully move on to the next stage. It is possible to think of the stages as a continuum in which the child establishes ego development features. This is a hierarchical structure in which each developmental issue is present in the previous stage and is further worked out in subsequent stages. A stage is presented as a duality with the usual outcome as a balance between the two extremes. As with any "stage," the reader needs to bear in mind that there are no distinct markers of stages and that the process of movement is not a straight line, as implied by the theoretical model. Cognitively, we like to have things nice and clearly delineated; nature doesn't always work that way. The process of ego maturation is a sloppy, meandering one that becomes hard to describe and to grasp intellectually.

Erikson's Eight Stages

Trust Versus Mistrust

At this first stage the infant must come to recognize that the world is basically a safe place—that needs are going to be met and that there is some consistency and order to the world. In order for the child to feel trust, the world must be predictable and the people who inhabit that world (mainly the primary caretaker) must be trustworthy and responsive in predictable and positive ways. It is believed that failure to develop this basic trust leads to the development of the severest forms of infantile schizophrenia.

Autonomy Versus Shame and Doubt

During this stage, the child develops a sense of personal power, of having some control over the world. This begins as some motor control is established, and as speech and language develop, the child can make wants known and begin to control others. Unfortunately, autonomy frequently emerges as a negative reaction to the desires of the parents: thus is born the "terrible two's." The child is working on establishing boundaries; the task of the parents is to help the child develop a sense of autonomy with a benign conscience. If the child is controlled by shame, he or she will tend to become an adult who governs by the letter rather than the spirit of the law and suffers from compulsive behavior.

Initiative Versus Guilt

In this stage, the child learns to be assertive, to take risks. The normal child moves into the larger adult society in an intrusive manner characterized by vigorous movements, and by occasional aggressiveness (especially toward siblings). There is also an insatiable curiosity manifested by the asking of endless questions. The task of the parents is to allow the child movement into the adult world without clamping down so much as to limit initiative. Too many restrictions by the parents cause the child to develop a highly constricted conscience based on guilt, which limits the child's willingness to risk. Psychopathology at this stage leads to an adult who exhibits hysterical denial, overconstricts self to the point of self-obliteration, or develops a great many psychosomatic diseases.

Industry Versus Inferiority

This stage coincides with the so-called latency period, generally when the child is between the ages of 5 and 11 years, although when one examines what occurs during this age span, it is clear that latency is a misnomer. Equipped with a sense of trust in the world and with some trust in self because of being allowed to develop autonomy and initiative, the child is now ready to learn formal skills. Society accommodates by providing the school in its many manifestations; here the technological fundamentals of the society are learned. The child acquires the tools that will be necessary in order to assume adulthood. The danger to the child at this stage is that a sense of adequacy may not develop, either through the failure of the family to prepare the child for school or the failure of the school to capitalize on the child's emerging abilities. An adult who has had difficulty at the industry level develops feelings of inadequacy compared with peers.

Identity Versus Role Confusion

Erikson's recognition of the adolescent experience as predominantly an issue of identity has received a great deal of attention and confirmation from developmental psychologists. The adolescent's task is to establish independence and freedom from the family and then, in the latter stages of adolescence, to establish a social role. The adolescent uses the parents as his or her first role model, and because the adolescent is also working on establishing independence from the family, will appoint the same-sex parent as the enemy. There is a time when the parents are a total embarrassment to the adolescent. This is especially true for the oldest child; subsequent children have two models to work from and they are usually easier for the parents to deal with as they fall somewhere between the extreme of the parents and the oldest sibling.

Establishment of identity is a very complex process because it is also heavily influenced by significant adults outside of the family: Other family members, teachers, neighbors, and even characters in plays and movies all influence the adolescent's search for identity. Children raised in single-parent homes must use these outside sources to help them establish identity.

Identity is actually accomplished through life experiences. As we encounter situations in which we have some success and some failure, we get a more rounded picture of ourselves. Identity, then, is a constantly evolving attribute as we go through the life cycle. Failure to establish an identity during adolescence leads to gender confusion and role confusion.

Intimacy Versus Isolation

Erikson was one of the first child analysts to recognize that the life cycle did not cease at adolescence but continued into adulthood. Adulthood is not static, but fraught with crises. As a child I often thought that when I was 30 I would "have it all together." I now recognize that growth is a continuous process: At times there are plateaus and at other times there are "breakup" periods; perhaps the times when we think we have it all together are just interludes to be enjoyed and savored.

At this stage, the young adult is an independent and self-governing individual; the task is to establish new ties to the world, free of the family relationships. These ties will evolve into the establishment of new primary relationships and of an occupation. Those adults who have a fragile sense of identity dare not enter into intimate relationships for fear of losing self, whereas those individuals who have little sense of self try to fuse with another and establish identity through the other person. In a truly intimate, loving relationship, both parties can and do maintain their separate identities. The young adult must find this balance—not an easy task.

Work also involves a fusion in which one must try to maintain a separate identity while feeling a part of the institution. An individual with a fragile ego becomes fearful of being swallowed by the institution and fails to commit, whereas an individual with little personal sense of identity will tend to overcommit and merge personal identity with work identity. Neither solution is healthy, and the failure to solve the intimacy crisis leads to a deep sense of isolation and alienation.

Generativity Versus Stagnation

This stage involves the need to ensure the existence of the species either by literally becoming a parent or by sharing knowledge and skills with the young. It is the life cycle stage that is characterized by productivity and creativity. This is the stage of altruism wherein adults forego their own personal needs to care for others. Generativity does not necessarily mean becoming a parent. One can figuratively instruct or care for future generations through work or charity. The mature human, according to Erikson, needs to instruct and teach. Thus is born the impulse to become a parent, write a book, compose a symphony, and so on.

The mere fact that one becomes a parent does not ensure that one has arrived at generativity. Some parents who have not resolved earlier issues around intimacy and identity are not able to give. They are still very self-absorbed and narcissistic, as one would expect at an earlier stage of ego development. In a similar vein, one's work can be long and strenuous but not very productive. Generativity enriches the individual as well as society; when such enrichment fails to take place, the individual stagnates.

Ego Integrity Versus Despair

For the aging or aged adult who has successfully negotiated the previous seven stages, this is the age of wisdom and detachment. It is the ability to see human problems in their entirety in the face of approaching death. One is able to love on a species-wide basis in the deepest sense. The mature elderly continue to grow and to adjust. The mature adult with ego integrity does not fear death and recognizes it as an integral part of the life cycle. Growing old does not guarantee that one will grow wise. There are elderly adults who fear death, who feel that life is now too short for them to engage in any new endeavor, and who are mired in despair.

Life Cycle and Communication Disorders

Use of the Erikson life cycle model in the field of communication disorders has not been extensive. I have found one detailed application of it; Schlessinger and Meadow (1971), in their study of deafness and mental health, used the Erikson model as a theory for explaining the discrepancy between the normal potential and the relatively poor achievement of deaf people. Using their clinical experience, they found the developmental framework provided by the life cycle model valuable in looking at the deaf child. It appears that at each life cycle stage, the deaf child has a more formidable task in resolving that particular crisis than does the normally hearing child.

One might assume that the development of basic trust may be impaired because of the delays and uncertainties in diagnosis of the deafness and the consequent anxiety of the parents. The parental grief reaction, which involves a great deal of anger and sorrow, also suggests that the deaf child may not receive the consistency of parental care and responsiveness that is vital to the development of trust. When the deaf infant is undergoing diagnosis, the world must seem a very frightening place with many strangers and many unexplained parental absences.

The lack of clear communication can limit the development of autonomy and initiative in a deaf child. For example, parents cannot explain why a rule is imposed, nor can the child ask the necessary questions to find out about the world. Parents also tend to limit their child physically because of the deafness, fearing that the child may not respond appropriately to danger. There is also high parental guilt, which is reflected in the attitude that "I let something bad happen to you once and I'm not about to let something bad happen to you again," and parents tend to overprotect.

At the competency level, the deaf child is again limited by the poor communication skills and the overprotection of teachers and parents. Much of our skill acquisition is dependent on explanations. Teacher expectation of deaf children as low achievers may also limit the competency of the deaf child, who also tends to internalize this judgment of the significant adults in the world.

Identity problems are particularly acute in the deaf child of hearing parents. In addition to the normal struggle to establish self, the deaf child has an apparent choice between the "hearing world" and the "deaf world." The child's problems are compounded if he or she has been raised orally, which too often involves a denial of deafness and the absence of a hearing-impaired peer group to relate to or any significant deaf adults to use as role models.

Schlessinger and Meadow (1971) observed that schools for the deaf have not equipped young deaf people properly for their introduction into the adult world. According to them, the young adult deaf person is not prepared to understand the intangible rules of the hearing society and frequently regresses to a more dependent status, much to the chagrin of teachers and parents. It is also hard for these young adults to develop a sense of generativity because of society's discrimination against the deaf. Love and work become very difficult under such conditions.

Almost nothing is known about the aged deaf; this is a largely unexplored area of investigation. One might assume that with the increased difficulty that they experience at each life cycle level, few deaf people achieve ego integrity; or if they do, they must travel a different route, one that is harder and more circuitous than that of the hearing population.

It would be very interesting to use the Erikson model on other populations with disabilities to see how they are affected; to my knowledge, this has not been done.

Life Cycle and Relationship Building

I have found the life cycle model to be a very useful way of looking at the development of a healthy counseling relationship, which is critical for growth. I find I can use this model at times to diagnose relationships that do not seem to be working—to find the point to which I need to return in order to develop a fruitful relationship. The life cycle notion helps us to understand how to build a relationship, as there seems to be a hierarchical function to relationship building similar to that in the life cycle model, in which each stage that is worked on has its origins in previous stages, and is worked out further in later stages.

Trust

Trust is the bedrock of a healthy relationship. Unfortunately, many professional relationships are not built on trust, and there can be no growth in relationships unless trust is present. There are three basic elements in building trust: caring, consistency, and credibility.

Caring is conveyed to the client in any number of ways, not the least of which is by active and sensitive listening. Kopp (1978), a psychotherapist, wrote,

> My first task was the creation of an atmosphere of trust within which we can enter into a therapeutic alliance. I begin by listening carefully to what a new patient has to say and to how it is said. I do not yet listen for the underlying dynamics that contribute to the patient's unhappiness. At the beginning, I am only trying to discover how it must feel to be that particular patient. For a while I do little more than try to formulate how the patient feels and to reflect those feelings back to the patient. It is enough that she finds that I am trying to understand how she experiences her life and that I help her to clarify her feelings without judging them. (p. 81)

The key to the notion of trust building is nonjudgmental listening. If someone is willing to try to hear my fears and my concerns and responds to my feelings without telling me that I "shouldn't feel that way," then I can be more open and trusting. Joysa Post (1983), a speech–language pathologist who had a stroke and became aphasic, found that the quality she responded to the most in the clinicians who worked with her was caring. She needed a clinician "who cared and was interested in me as a person" (p. 23).

Trust develops when one believes that the people are reliable. This is shown by the very simple things that clinicians can do. I start meetings on time and always end them when we have agreed to end them. If I cannot be at a meeting, I warn the clients ahead of time. If I have misrepresented issues or erred in some way, I apologize and correct the error. I try to be transparent about my feelings and my concerns. I also never tell clients anything that I cannot verify.

In the initial stages of relationship, we are granted credibility by virtue of title. We give trust to someone who bears the title "doctor" (especially if a white coat is worn). Over time, however, credibility has to be earned. In part we earn it by what we know and how we convey it. The information given by the professional early in diagnosis is seldom retained by the clients because affect is so high. What is being worked on without either party being aware of it is the establishment of credibility. I will trust a professional if I think he or she knows the field even if at that point I do not have a sufficient corpus of stored information to evaluate the information being provided.

There are also all the intangibles of credibility establishment, which are conveyed to others by how I conduct myself, whether I seem to be in control of myself, and whether I share my information. Oddly enough, I have found that I do not lose credibility—in fact I gain it—when I am willing to tell clients that I do not know something. They are then willing to trust the other information that I provide. My willingness to tag something as unknown by me gives them the confidence to believe that what I do say is known. (Of course, there are times when what I think is "known" is not a fact; too many of these, and I lose all credibility. It is my professional responsibility to keep my information up-to-date.)

One of the surest ways to lose credibility is by reassurance. Although the people we are dealing with frequently seek reassurance, when we give it, we also diminish ourselves. When we tell people that it will be okay in order to help make them feel better, they know that we cannot know that it will be better, and we lose credibility. I am always suspicious of anyone who seems to be telling me what I want to hear: At one level it is soothing; at another, though, I lose trust in what the person is telling me.

Autonomy

Autonomy in a relationship is control that each party has; it is the feeling that I can make things happen that I perceive are in my best interest. Autonomy is always established in relationship to someone else; it is a bouncing-off that requires some form of negotiation with someone else, usually someone who is perceived as being more powerful. When the powerful other is the parent, then the child must be given some sense of control—some choices that are respected by the adult. This can save a great deal of grief. I remember walking one time with my four-year-old daughter at a fair, and it was quite clear we were both getting fatigued. I suggested to her that she sit down, and since she was working on autonomy in a big way at that time, her only possible response was "no." My wife, standing next to me, turned to her and said, "Alison, which chair are you going to sit on, the red one or the blue one?" and Alison promptly sat: She now had some control. She was permitted a choice and her choice was respected. We all need that sense of control in our relationships.

Often the powerful other in relationships is the professional. How much autonomy do we allow in therapy? My observation of most therapy is that very little autonomy is granted to the client. I think this comes about as a result of the "lesson plan syndrome." Students in training are expected to enter therapy with specific plans and goals. This gives the therapist, especially the insecure beginning therapist, control of the situation. More experienced therapists will be flexible and modify a plan depending on the client. How many therapists, I wonder, develop the lesson plans in conjunction with the specific client, where both sit down and decide the agenda for that meeting? Autonomy can be encouraged in such little ways as, for example, the audiologist asking the client after a diagnostic evaluation, "What do you need to know?" rather than delivering a set speech and making all the decisions regarding the kind of information needed.

The professional has difficulty giving autonomy to the client on two counts, the first of which is the time element. When there is a waiting room full of patients, it is much more expedient to give the set speech and send the client out the door. This expeditious solution is usually the least efficient on a long-term basis, however, because the set speech is rarely retained and the client will generally return with the same lack of knowledge. What I do with clients is tell them, "I have 15 minutes [or whatever time I do have available]. How would you like to use this time?"

Second, the professional is worried that "they might not ask the right question." In the context of a counseling relationship, there are no wrong questions. Generally, if clients do not ask the question, they are not ready to hear the answer, and the information provided is seldom digested. People will learn only what they are ready to learn and absorb. The best indication of readiness is the question: Gratuitous information usually serves to increase confusion and is rarely helpful. There are times when it is appropriate for us as professionals to provide information without being asked, and when this device is successful, it is generally because we have responded to the unasked question, which first requires sensitive listening.

Initiative

Initiative is an element of relationships that is very closely related to autonomy. Initiative is the positive side of autonomy. Autonomy usually is established by the "no" in relationship to the powerful other and in some ways is easier than taking the initiative because the person does not have to take responsibility for his or her behavior. It is much easier to know what is not wanted than to take the responsibility for getting what is wanted. Initiative is fostered by the professional leaving spaces—teaching by creating vacuums. If I do not take total responsibility for what is going on, then the other person in the relationship has to act. It may seem damaging to my professional ego, but often the less I do, the more the other person learns in the relationship. This means that we are going to have to change some of the definitions of professional responsibility. So often the professional must "do" in order to satisfy the job description and the supervisors, while listening and responding are not always seen by either the therapist or the supervisor as being effective professional behavior. We need to change this attitude. Professionals are going to have to learn to be comfortable with silences and with "not doing" so as to create spaces in which the client can take initiative. We grow through the acceptance of responsibility balanced by self-protection. Clients must learn to achieve this balance, and clinicians must help them in this task.

There are some dangers in this approach to fostering initiative. For one, we will violate the client's expectation of what a professional should do. (The client may ask, "Why am I paying you?") This violation will generate anger, which may or may not surface, that if not dealt with, can distort the relationship. The anger itself is a marvelous spur to taking initiative on the client's part, if the clinician can sensitively handle it. Second, if we do not act, we may lose credibility; there is a fine line that the professional must very delicately tread. The difference for me is in being responsible *to* (or responsive to) the clients rather than being responsible *for* them. Although I try to do 50% of the work and invite the other person to do his or her 50%, it is often hard to locate the therapeutic equator of responsibility.

Autonomy and initiative are attributes that are especially important for parents of children with disabilities to develop. They will need these traits in devising educational plans for their children in conjunction with the public school professionals. It is very easy for the parents to be intimidated by the confrontation with professionals. By now it should also be clear to the reader that initiative and autonomy are "loci of control" issues. Inner locus of control is obtained through the development of initiative and autonomy. (This issue will be discussed in more detail in Chapter 6.)

Industry

Industry is the relationship level at which most professionals seem to relate to their clients. There is clearly a task to be accomplished: a communication disorder to be overcome, a deaf child to be educated, a hearing aid to be obtained. Unfortunately, most professionals are so content or problem centered that they ignore the issues of trust, autonomy, and initiative. The professional anxiety to alleviate the problem gets in the way of the establishment of the necessary precursors to effective joint work. The therapeutic alliance is not established when the professionals do much more than their 50%, and they often begin to complain about lack of client motivation.

Learning is obtained by any of three routes: by being told (lecture), by seeing (demonstration), and by doing. The most lasting way of learning is by doing. Unfortunately, for parent groups, in particular, the professionals seem to use the lecture as the primary learning vehicle. Many parent discussion groups are really lectures provided by the professional on some topic that may or may not have been selected by the parent group. A lecture is a very inefficient way to teach because it assumes, incorrectly, that the audience is homogeneous in knowledge. The degree to which the learners have developed some trust will be reflected in their willingness to ask questions and take some initiative for their own learning. It is often difficult to get parents to ask questions after a lecture, when there is a low level of trust in the group.

As a teaching device, demonstration is very tricky. If it is not used sensitively, it can deskill the learner by increasing feelings of incompetency. I saw this occur in an itinerant therapy program when I worked with both the teachers and the parents of young deaf children. In this program, the teacher had to travel several hours to get to the parents' home and she had only a limited time to spend with the child. The teacher often brought in the child's favorite toy and invariably gave a successful lesson. The child was generally very eager to see the teacher as she came only once a week and always had a new toy to play with, which she used skillfully. The lesson almost always went well and the therapist would then tell the parent who was observing to continue working on this lesson during the week. When the parent tried to do the lesson by imitating what she had seen the therapist do, however, she usually failed. The failure occurred for a variety of reasons: The child was too familiar with the parent and resented the parent as teacher; the parent had many emotional issues about the child and often was not able to see the child clearly; and the parent was probably not very competent (why should she be?), which is why she was in the program in the first place. In itinerant programs of this sort, the parent is almost always programmed for failure, and thus begins to feel even more incompetent.

My own bias about itinerant programs is that they should be entirely parent centered. I think that the teacher needs to see the parent as the recipient of the teaching and should rarely work directly with the child.

A similar loss of competency can occur when the supervisor demonstrates to the student clinician a more effective way to establish the desired behavior in a client. This demonstration usually is done easily and effortlessly by the supervisor and leaves the student feeling totally incompetent. The supervisor who then goes to a conference and observes a master clinician at work may also feel incompetent. Demonstration, if not done sensitively, can have the opposite of the intended effect and leave the learner in worse shape. This is not to say demonstration does not have a place in teaching; it can be a very valuable tool when there is enough trust in the relationship and when the learner already has established some self-esteem.

Doing is by far the most efficient way to learn, especially if one has a sensitive supervisor–teacher observing. Doing requires the highest degree of trust, for no one likes to appear incompetent, and the learner, by definition, is supposed to be incompetent. In order to learn, the student must be willing to reveal areas of ignorance to the teacher. Unfortunately, most educational programs reward competency and penalize ignorance; therefore, students learn to try to please the teacher by guessing what is in the teacher's head and by trying to appear competent when they are not.

Holt (1964) noticed that elementary school children, when given the task of trying to guess a number, would be disturbed by a "no" answer despite the fact that they gained as much information from a "no" answer as they did from a "yes." He concluded that one of the reasons children fail is because they are afraid of failure. No initiative can be taken unless there is a willingness to be wrong. In order for effective learning to take place, we must remove all penalty for failure and we must encourage mistakes (to put that another way, we must encourage learners to take risks). I have learned far more from my mistakes than I have from my successes. The failure tells me where my limit is and where I need to learn more. My successes, while gratifying, reflect skills that I have already mastered and no longer need to learn.

The unconditional regard, the caring that I convey to the learners, allows them to take risks. In short, there must be trust present for skills to be taught and learned. Each of these techniques of lecturing, demonstrating, and doing has a value in learning, and, in a particular time and place, each one may be appropriate. As we shall see in the next chapter, timing is all important.

Identity

Identity is very much role dependent; that is, how I define myself and how others define me will determine my behavior to a large degree. It is a function of the expectations that I and others have for that particular role. It is very easy to become role bound.

For example, the role of the "parent" has a connotation for someone who is not really involved in the educational or therapeutic process of the child. I remember once waiting outside my child's school to pick her up after an extracurricular activity. The principal, who did not know me, was concerned about a man lurking near the school. He asked me who I was, and I responded, "I am just a parent." Without skipping a beat, he responded, "What do you mean, *just* a parent?" We discussed that issue at length. Parents, as they usually define themselves in relationship to school, are an appendage of their child, someone who provides transportation, supplies, and lunch money, and who attends PTA meetings to be told things about their child. They are always on the periphery of things and not really important to the learning process that is taking place in the school.

The role of "patient" also has a connotation of passivity, which is precisely why I have used the word *client* rather than *patient* throughout this text. The whole process of becoming a patient involves losing individuality. A patient goes to the doctor, receives a prescription, and follows it in order to get well. In a hospital setting, the patient is expected to be a very passive part of the process while the professionals do the work. When patients refuse to cooperate—that is, conform to the role expectation—the doctors and nurses are immensely disturbed. Lear's (1980) book *Heartsounds* gives a remarkable view of the patient process from someone who has seen it from the physician's perspective. Her husband, a physician, found that when he became a heart patient the attending physicians stopped listening to him and began treating him as a disease rather than as a person. His first act in recovering from his heart attack was to stop wearing the hospital johnny coat in order to retrieve some of his personhood.

The holistic health movement, which seems to be gaining more respect these days, puts the patients at the center of the healing process and requires them to take some responsibility for the course of therapy. I hope that this trend will continue in medical practice.

Probably the most role-bound individual in the therapeutic process is the professional. He or she usually is defined as the person who has the knowledge and the skill to make the other person "better"; therefore, the professional has the responsibility for making things happen, in short for being "smart" and having the answers. Professionals are expected to write prescriptions and give advice. The manner of dress is usually very narrowly prescribed (in some settings, it has to be a white coat) and the terms of address are carefully spelled out—usually with a formality that keeps a patient–therapist distance. Most of this self-protective behavior is taught at the training level and is readily adopted by the student clinician. A fully defined role is a means of gaining security: If one knows exactly what is expected, then one can conform to those expectations and behave appropriately. The price one pays for this security is a rigidity in behavior that may very well limit growth. In fact, very often the traditional patient–therapist relationship has many features that limit the development of a healthy relationship; in particular, it fails in the responsibility assumption area because the locus of control is external to the patient and in the hands of the therapist.

In the wholesome counseling relationship, where there are high levels of trust, where both parties are free to take initiative and have retained their autonomy, and where role definitions are not rigid, it might be very hard for the casual observer to decide who is the professional and who is the client.

Intimacy

Intimacy is very much tied to trust. When a high level of trust exists in a relationship, we can risk being open. Openness leads to a sense of caring and closeness. Intimacy also involves risk: The fear of intimacy often manifests itself in personally distancing behavior, which is often self-defeating.

In a counseling relationship, both parties need to feel that they can say what needs to be said. Only what is important between them is discussed and revealed. I do not have to disclose my bank balance in order to be intimate; however, when appropriate, I do need to relate—either verbally or nonverbally—how I feel about the other person. There is surety in knowing how the other person in a relationship is feeling. Intimacy also involves negative feelings. A great deal of trust is required before I can reveal that I am angry. Professionals who are role bound often feel that they do not have the right to be angry at clients. This attitude severely limits intimacy because no true intimacy is possible unless the full range of feelings that exist in a relationship can be expressed.

Intimacy carries with it the possibility of pain. As I become more caring and closer to people, I also leave myself vulnerable to loss when the relationship ends. Because of the anticipated pain of separation, many people limit their closeness. The price of this solution is an interpersonal loneliness. Here again, each of us must make a personal choice and resolve the interpersonal dilemma for ourself. Teaching—and, by extension, clinical work—is a very painful profession because many of our relationships are clearly limited in duration. The professional's temptation to limit intimacy and pain is therefore very great, which means that we do not develop relationships that have maximum growth possibilities. I have found that when I limit risks, I also limit gains; hence, I have chosen to develop close relationships. The price I pay in June when both students and parents depart is well worth the joy I have experienced during the semester. No relationships are permanent; therefore, I want to and choose to extract the most from each relationship that I have.

Generativity

Generativity becomes the outward manifestation of the skills learned during the industry phase. Now the client can go beyond the therapeutic relationship to demonstrate and develop increased skills in other relationships. This becomes the therapeutic carryover issue.

Out of the successful therapeutic relationship should also come the impulse toward altruism—toward making things better for others. It is no accident that many of our speech pathologists were themselves at one time recipients of therapy. Although this might also reflect an identity issue, very often it is a reflection of the desire to give to others something of value that has been received. This is the noblest human drive.

I have watched parents go through the grieving process; they generally tend to progress from concern about themselves to concern about their child, and finally to concern about all deaf children. Parents are potentially a major resource for change, and the desire to help others can be channeled by the clinician to provide huge benefits to the community. Parents can and do become very active in promoting legislation and prodding bureaucrats to do the things that they should be doing. This very fruitful energy arises from a healthy therapeutic relationship that grows into the generativity or productivity stage.

Integrity

Integrity is the terminal phase of the relationship. Our job as therapists and teachers is to do ourselves out of our job, to no longer be needed. We are not doing our job well if we cannot let go of the clients we are serving, and, although this is painful, termination needs to be recognized as a necessary part of the therapeutic cycle.

Because of my own death avoidance issues, I once tried to keep termination discussion in my relationships to an absolute minimum. I came to see that this was a mistake. There is a need to "close up shop," take a detached view of the relationship, and process the experience. There is a need to bring the relationship to closure, to explain why I did or did not do certain things, to talk about previously concealed feelings, and to express often latent feelings of appreciation. I usually feel a sense of sadness at this time and a sense of loss. When I think about the new relationships that will be starting in the fall, I feel a momentary sense of despair at having to start the process over again. I wonder if the new relationships will be as satisfying. I also feel some excitement at the prospect of encountering new people and learning something more about myself.

Models as Clinical Tools

Models can be very dangerous if taken literally by the unwary reader, because they are a simplification of a very complex process. It might seem from reading this chapter that relationship building proceeds smoothly through the eight outlined stages, and that if a relationship is stuck, then all one has to do to diagnose the trouble is go back to the sticking point. In practice, this is not so simple: Relationship building is at best a sloppy process with different stages being worked on at different times, not necessarily sequentially. At times, some issues are only partially worked out and then returned to; very often, several stages are being worked on simultaneously.

Models become clinically valuable as conceptualizations; they enable us to talk about very complex phenomena by giving us a vocabulary. The reader must always bear in mind that the model is a simplification and not the event—it is but a particular abstraction of an event.

I have found the existential model and the Erikson life cycle model to be particularly helpful clinically. They complement one another nicely. The existential view focuses on current behavior that seems to be universal, whereas the Erikson model gives a developmental perspective within our culture. There are large areas of overlap between them; for example, the Erikson stages of autonomy and initiative are comparable to the existential issue of responsibility assumption; identity and productivity are intricately related to the meaning issue; trust and intimacy are very much part of the loneliness experience; and of course death is part and parcel of the ego integrity stage.

Despite the overlap, these models give us somewhat different views of human beings, and we can use whichever conceptualization seems most appropriate for describing a particular behavior. The reader must always bear in mind that there is no "right" view of human behavior—only a variety of ways to interpret a particular facet of behavior.

4

The Emotions
of Communication
Disorders

To have a communication disorder is also to have strong feelings; this is true for both the client and the family of the client. Communication is so basic to humanness that when it is blocked or distorted we become emotionally upset. Often the display of feelings is very distressing to the speech and hearing professional, in part, I think because of the lack of training in affect counseling. For most professionals in our field, there is an underlying supposition that the people we encounter are so emotionally fragile that any mistake on our part might send them over the edge. This makes us professionals wary in exposing our own and our client's feelings. As a beginning audiologist, I think I tried to forestall emotional displays because I was embarrassed by them and because I did not know how to react appropriately; I also felt vaguely guilty that I had somehow caused the pain, and in some ways I had, by being the bearer of bad news.

My difficulty in handling affect with my clients (as well as in my personal life) led me to employ all sorts of strategies to prevent feelings from emerging. I often used my sense of humor as a distraction designed to try to make people feel better. Alternatively, as a principal distraction, I provided information to keep people in their cognitive realm and away from feelings. I have learned, however, that the goal of counseling is not to make people feel better, but to separate feelings from nonproductive behavior. The feelings must always be acknowledged. I also have found that people have many diverse ways to make themselves feel better and I can just allow that to happen; they were not really so fragile as I had assumed.

It is always a mistake in any relationship to tell people, no matter how nicely we do it, that they shouldn't feel a particular way. When we do this, we help them to feel guilty about their feelings, as though they should not have them. Probably the least helpful thing to say to anybody is, "Don't worry about it," because then they start worrying about their worrying. What we really mean by "don't worry" or "don't feel that way" is that "your expression of feelings is distressing to me so please stop." It is hard to see how this strategy can ever be helpful to people we want to help.

The operative rule for the counseling model described in this book is that feelings are neither good nor bad; they just are. They need to be acknowledged and accepted, but not judged. There is deep pain in having a communication disorder, and in many cases we cannot do or say anything that will take the pain away. It needs to be acknowledged for what it is, a very normal reaction to a terrible situation. Behavior, on the other hand, can be judged. We can see whether it is self-enhancing, that is, whether it is accomplishing the goals we would like it to accomplish. If it isn't, we can set about changing it.

This chapter describes the feelings associated with the catastrophic changes in families that are commonly seen by speech and hearing professionals. We examine the feelings and look at the behaviors that arise from these feelings. Behaviors confound the therapist–client relationship if the therapist does not understand the affective source of the behavior. I have found in my work with a very diverse population that affect is universal, at least to our culture, and is not disorder specific. We as a species tend to respond in the same way to catastrophic events in our lives. The display of the emotions is unique to each individual and the content is unique to each disorder, but the grief process is the same. It is always a sense of loss.

Grief

In all change there is a loss. For anyone undergoing catastrophic change, it is the loss of the expected future that is grieved so deeply. For my wife and me, it is the loss of how we envisioned ourselves after our children left home. (They all have left now.) Instead of having a very vigorous middle age, with many trips and lots of hiking and running, which we both like to do, the reality is her disability; we never planned on my wife's being in a wheelchair. There is always pain for the loss, and it is a pain that never leaves you. One father of a deaf child said, "When you first find out your child is deaf, it hurts like hell. Then it becomes a dull ache that never goes away." The pain of that loss never goes away—and it is not our role to take that pain away. Rather, as one mother of a deaf child said, "I have the same feelings but they no longer control me."

The process of coming to grips with this loss is much like the response to a death because it is the death of a dream or an expectation. Much of the monumental work of Kubler-Ross (1969) in her astute observations of the terminally ill and dying is applicable to the losses experienced by persons with communication disorders and their families. However, I have found Kubler-Ross's stages of grief—denial, anger, bargaining, depression, and acceptance—a bit overused and too simplistic for a very complex process.

I am always leery of any "stages" concept in the grief process. I think the process is basically amorphous, having fluid boundaries and being cyclical in nature rather than being a straight-line progression, as implied by many models of the process. Featherstone (1980), the mother of a child with severe disabilities, described the grief process so well when she wrote,

> But I am uncomfortable with most stage theories, they carry too heavy a freight of straight line progress; they also suggest an implausible final harmony. The actual progress is not linear, and often is bought at a high price in human suffering. In the vocabulary of stages, acceptance becomes a kind of high plateau, once out of reach, now firmly felt underfoot. Gone are the fears and self-reproaches of yesterday and sighs for what might have been. Matter of fact realism guides our effort. Having struggled out of darkness, we will not have to be afraid anymore. . . . Few parents reach an emotional promised land; most have good days and bad days. (p. 232)

Tanner (1980) wrote a comprehensive article on the grief reaction and how this relates to the speech pathologist/audiologist. He commented that loss can be both real and symbolic, and that grief is not a single reaction but a complex progression involving many emotions and attempts to cope with loss. I find it clinically more profitable to examine the feelings in loss rather than seek the stages of mourning.

Behaviorally, the bereaved can get stuck in their loss and not see what is there for them because they are so busy mourning what they have lost. I recently came across the following piece, which I use in parent groups to help facilitate the grief process:

> When you're going to have a baby, it's like planning a wonderful vacation trip to Italy. You get a bunch of guide books and make all your plans. The Coliseum . . . the Michelangelo David . . . the gondolas in Venice. You get a book of handy phrases and learn how to say a few words in Italian. It's all very exciting.

Finally, the time comes for your trip. You pack your bags and off you go.

Several hours later, the plane lands. The stewardess comes in and says, "Welcome to Holland."

"Holland?!?" you say. "Holland?? I signed up for Italy! All my life I've dreamed of going to Italy!"

"I'm sorry," she says. "There's been a change and we've landed in Holland."

"But I don't know anything about Holland! I never thought of going to Holland. I have no idea what you do in Holland!"

What's important is that they haven't taken you to a terrible ugly place, full of famine, pestilence and disease. It's just—a *different* place.

So you have to go out and buy a whole new set of guide books . . . you have to learn a whole new language . . . and you'll meet a whole new bunch of people you would never have met otherwise.

Holland. It's slower-paced than Italy, less flashy than Italy . . . but after you've been there for a while, and you've had a chance to catch your breath, you look around and begin to discover that Holland has windmills . . . and Holland has tulips . . . Holland even has Rembrandts.

But everyone you know is busy coming and going from Italy . . . and they're all bragging about what a great time they had there. And for the rest of your life you will say, "Yes, that's where I was supposed to go. That's what I had planned." And the pain of that will never, ever, ever, ever go away. And you must accept that pain—because the loss of that dream is a very very significant loss.

But . . . if you spend your time mourning the fact that you never got to go to Italy, you may never be available to enjoy the very *lovely*, very *special* things about Holland."

(Emily Perle Kinsley; used with permission)

So many mourners feel stuck in "Holland"—always bemoaning the fact that they are not in "Italy." The ultimate goal of counseling, as I see it, is to help people recognize what Holland has to offer, and although they may always regret the lost trip to Italy, they can learn to appreciate what they have in Holland.

Feelings of Inadequacy

Anyone faced with a daunting change in life will experience feelings of being overwhelmed by and inadequate to deal with the new challenges posed by the catastrophic event. Parents of children with disabilities in particular feel overwhelmed. The responsibility is awesome. When parents are told that their child has a disability—a statement usually accompanied by an admonition of some helping professionals that "if this child is to succeed, then it is up to the parents"—the normal terror of parenthood is increased fourfold.

A direct concomitant of the feeling of being overwhelmed is the desire to be rescued. The rescue notion, on the parents' part, manifests itself in many ways. A frequent fantasy that emerges in parent support groups is, "Wouldn't it be nice if someone came and took my child and brought him back when he was 18, all civilized and talking beautifully!" This fantasy is usually presented with a laugh, but it does reflect the underlying insecurity and inadequacy felt by the parents. (This is also the appeal of the residential school that will take the responsibility from the parents.)

In one parent group, a father beseeched me to be the quarterback of his team. When I declined, he offered me the position of coach, which I also declined. The only role in his personal odyssey that I was willing to accept was that of enthusiastic fan. I told him that I would be in the stands, rooting hard and sharing all my information, but that he would have to select and send in his own plays.

When the professional calls the plays, the parents become the spectators and assume no responsibility for the outcome. They may either praise or blame the coach, but they are not involved. Spectators seldom grow or learn very much.

Unfortunately, too many professionals in our field are willing to call the plays (see, e.g., the Dee, 1981, article cited in Chapter 1). It is a very difficult trap to avoid. The people whom we are pledged to help are coming to us in a great deal of pain and are feeling inadequate and overwhelmed by the responsibility. They often say, "I'm just a parent; you're the professional." Since we have a great deal of information and compassion, it is tempting to take the responsibility from the parents and rescue them. To do so, however, creates spectators of the parents (or anyone else facing a marked life change).

Probably the best example in contemporary literature of the ultimate rescuer is in the story of Annie Sullivan and Helen Keller. Annie Sullivan, especially as depicted in the film *The Miracle Worker,* became a role model and a vocational inspiration for many in our profession. A biography written by Lash (1980) gives a more complete story of the Annie Sullivan–Mrs. Keller–Helen Keller triangle. Annie Sullivan had a very deprived childhood. After her mother's death, the six-year-old Annie and her four-year-old brother were placed in a home for the indigent by their alcoholic father. Her brother died shortly after being placed in the facility, and Annie literally had nothing while growing up among destitute, elderly people. Because of a visual problem, she was sent to the Perkins School for the Blind in Boston and received her education among an institutionalized blind population. The plea for help from the Kellers arrived as Annie was graduating, and she was sent to Alabama to rescue the family. It is easy to imagine the young Annie Sullivan as a descending angel or, to use a storybook character, Mary

Poppins. She must at least have seemed this way to the desperate Kellers, who had an out-of-control, deaf–blind child.

There is a scene in the movie that represents a professional climax. Shortly after arriving at the Kellers' home, Annie was to be introduced to her charge at a formal Sunday afternoon dinner. Annie was waiting at the fully laden table with Helen's father and brother. Mrs. Keller entered with Helen, and it was very apparent that she had no control over the child. Helen was making gruesome noises and totally disrupted the meal by throwing food. The father and brother left in a huff, and Mrs. Keller looked across the table to Annie in total despair.

At this point, Annie had a choice to make: to work with Mrs. Keller and teach her how to manage her child or to rescue Mrs. Keller by taking the child. If Annie had worked with Mrs. Keller, then Annie would not have become famous and would not have received the credit. Mrs. Keller might have! For Annie to have done this, she would have to have had what psychologists call an "inner locus of evaluation," the ability to pat oneself on the back and let others get the credit. To do this, one has to be a reasonably congruent person. Annie, given her deprived childhood and her very strong need to be needed, chose to take Helen to a shack on the property and literally strapped Helen to her at night. Within two weeks she emerged with a civilized child who was beginning to communicate—a miracle! Since all of the viewers of the movie know that Helen turned out to be a truly remarkable deaf–blind person who achieved a great deal despite her disability, it is tempting to conclude that they lived happily ever after.

The Lash biography, however, continues the story. The effect on Mrs. Keller was profound. In a short time, Annie had accomplished more than Mrs. Keller had in the previous six years of trying to work with the child on her own. She was profoundly grateful, but at the same time more convinced than ever that she was an inadequate mother for such a child. After all, she could not work "miracles" the way Annie could. Mrs. Keller abandoned any further attempts to actively mother Helen and thereafter seemed to be reduced to the role of loving aunt.

Helen and Annie went back to Boston and achieved all the outward manifestations of success, including graduating from Radcliffe College. However, the closely dependent relationship that developed between them, in which Annie had almost all the control, could not work in Helen's best interest (or in Annie's). The goal of teaching, like the goal of parenting, is to encourage the child to be independent. Annie could not do this because she had so many needs to be needed that had not been fulfilled in her life. In many ways, she needed Helen more than Helen needed her. After Annie's death, Helen went through a succession of paid companions, none of whom satisfied her in the way that Annie did. She never learned how to live independently despite her formidable and remarkable skills.

The Annie Sullivan story is an extreme example of the rescue syndrome. Sometimes the most helpful thing we can do for our clients is to not help, or at least to not help in an overt manner. Often I have been much more useful to people who left my office saying, "Why did we go there? We knew all of that before we went," than if they have left saying, "What would we ever do without him?" We work in a helping profession, but to be truly helpful, our goal must be to enhance the self-esteem of our clients and their families. Overt assistance, although often appreciated, is also a statement that the recipient is inadequate and needs aid. Very often the overt aid leads to resentment on the recipient's part and also to diminished self-confidence. To nurture effectively is to give help in a sensitive, timely fashion that may not always be seen or appreciated by the recipient. We as professionals need to remain very much aware of our own needs to be needed, and to be able to pat ourselves on the back so that others may take the credit. Our goal in helping is to create independent people who no longer need help.

Anger

Almost anyone experiencing a catastrophic change will experience some anger. The person might not be aware of this anger and might not be able to express it, but it is there nonetheless. Anger has many sources, the predominant one being when there is a violation of expectations. At a very simple level, if you and I have an agreement to meet and you fail to show up, I will be very angry: It is a self-righteous anger. All parents have many expectations about their unborn child, most significantly that he or she will be normal. When the child is "defective," the parents are angry; they feel cheated.

Another expectation, doomed to failure, is that the disorder can be cured. Parents find it harder to accept the fact that there is no cure than to accept the fact that the child has a disability. (They say, for example, "We spend so much money to send an astronaut to the moon; why can't we find a cure for cerebral palsy?") The clients also have expectations of the professional and usually expect to be taken care of à la Annie Sullivan. (They saw the movie *The Miracle Worker*, too.) This expectation may or may not be violated.

The most pervasive, and perhaps most harmful, expectation that clients have is the idealized image of how they should perform. This expectation is fed by a steady stream of sitcom families on TV who resolve crises easily and with apparent calmness. This sets up an expectation in clients and their families that they, too, should be able to manage the change with a minimum of stress and pain. When this is not the case, they feel angry at themselves for being so "incompetent" and "weak." They are not able to see the reality that they are quite normal. This self-directed anger is very harmful, often manifesting itself as depression and low self-esteem.

Dealing with or having a communication disorder causes a loss of some personal freedom, which becomes another source of anger. When disability is present, our life options are narrowed and we get very angry at these restrictions. We have lost control of our lives. A father of a deaf child, for example, said,

> I have been working for several years to get a promotion in my company. I have wanted this very badly and today I was informed that I have the promotion. If I take it, though, it means that we will have to move to a small town which has no services for the deaf, and my son will have to go to a school for the deaf on a residential basis. My wife and I consider this option terrible. So now if I take the promotion I will screw up my son, and if I don't I will damage my career. I am very angry and frustrated!

This father's anger is very typical, as is the frustration of many mothers who decide to stay home to take care of their disabled children with disabilities and to forego their career advancements. Spouses, too, must make adjustments in their life plans because of the illness of their husbands or wives. The corporate executive, for example, who can no longer function at meetings because of his progressive hearing loss will be very angry and resentful. His wife will also be angry at the restrictions in their social life and perhaps at her being relegated to the role of, in the words of one wife, "a hearing ear dog." These are changes that are forced from the outside and over which people have little or no control. A loss of control always involves a great deal of anger.

Another source of the anger, which is more like rage, is the parent's or spouse's frustration over having a loved one hurting in some way and the inability to make it better for them. This feeling of impotence or powerlessness is devastating for me as I watch my wife stagger from one place to another and I'm unable to make things better for her. All parents are pledged to make things better for their children; when they cannot, they feel a terrible impotence that manifests itself as rage. Fathers and husbands are more likely to experience this kind of anger because of their family role. Men traditionally are the family protectors. Their job is to stand at the gates and slay any dragons that might be assaulting the family. When family members are hurting, the father feels he has failed, and he becomes frustrated and angry. In women, the anger traditionally tends to be turned inward, becoming depression; in men it usually gets displaced.

I think most professionals in our field recognize at some level that they are dealing with angry people. Many of the emotional distancing strategies employed—for example, keeping the relationship content based—are designed to keep at bay the eruption of the client volcano. Very often, client anger is displaced onto the professional, and the professional can easily become the lightning rod. People sometimes slay the messenger when they do not like the message.

Anger is a very difficult emotion in most relationships; it frequently is equated with loss of love. Most families do not have good strategies for dealing with anger other than to suppress it. It is usually seen as something very threatening to relationships and thus is often displaced onto innocent victims (dogs, cats, professionals) or turned inward to become depression.

When anger is subverted and not allowed to emerge, it poisons relationships. A person who is angry with me and does not tell me frequently operates in subversive ways. For example, the angry client chronically misses appointments, is bothered by very minor things such as the decor of the room or the comfort of the chair, and does not fully participate in the therapy. Unless I can tap into that anger and deal with it, the relationship will never be mutually satisfactory. If professionals do not deal well with their own anger, they become poor role models for their clients. Very often, professionals feel that they do not have the right to be angry with clients. How very demeaning this is to clients, because it also says, "You don't mean enough to me to provoke anger in me." Professionals will do many of the same things clients do in repressing and displacing their anger, thereby confounding the therapeutic relationship. Unexpressed anger is like a loaded cannon loose on deck that can go off at any moment and sink the vessel.

The source of much client–professional anger is implicit, unfulfilled expectations. In any relationship that has any degree of intimacy, the parties have expectations of themselves, of each other, and of the relationship. In a healthy relationship, almost all the expectations are made explicit so that if there is a violation of an explicit expectation, it can be dealt with in the course of the relationship. Less healthy relationships, and ultimately less stable ones, have many implicit expectations. These are the ones we assume the other person is going to fulfill, but we never express them to make them explicit. When these expectations are violated, we get angry; if we have not been explicit about our expectations, we cannot be direct about our anger, either.

For example, I may wake up in the morning wanting to have pasta for dinner, only I do not bother to tell my wife (I figure she loves me so much and we have been married so long that she should be able to read my mind). So I go off to work expecting pasta for supper. When I return home, because my wife is not always accurate in her mindreading, I get something else for dinner, which under ordinary circumstances would be delicious, but I get angry because it is not pasta. (The reader will recognize here the Italy/Holland issue in another guise.) Because I know that I did not ask for pasta in the morning, I know I do not have a right to complain about the lack of pasta at night; that, however, does not stop me from feeling angry. Because I know I cannot be overt about the anger because it would not be fair, I wait for my wife to do something annoying that under ordinary circumstances I might ignore. If she drops a cup or bites her fingernail while I am carrying this load of unexpressed anger, I zap her, and we have a big fight about the broken cup when I am really angry about the pasta. As long as we continue to fight about the cup our relationship makes no progress. Relationships can stand only so much of this before they crumble from the assaults of unfair anger.

Many professional–client relationships have failed because of implicit, unfulfilled expectations. Many expectations revolve, for example, around responsibility assumptions. The teacher/therapist may assume that the parent will be doing homework with the child, and the parent may assume that schoolwork is the province of the teacher. The undiscussed expectations lead to anger that is seldom expressed directly. The teacher/therapist and the parent need to discuss their mutual expectations, and a contract made. Then if there is a failed expectation, the anger can be expressed directly and the contract renegotiated if necessary.

It is not the implicit expectations per se that are the problems (although it always helps to make explicit that which is implicit and see if there is a match on expectations); it is the unwillingness to be direct about the anger that defeats relationships. Anger can be a very healthy emotion in relationships. Because there is a great deal of caring and energy in anger, it becomes the fuel of change. If clients are angry at me, I examine the anger to see if it is justified. If I have been derelict in my duty, I apologize and make amends if possible. If we are dealing with a situation in which there has been an implicit expectation that I have failed to meet, the anger then becomes an opportunity to clarify our relationship and make the expectations explicit. If I am dealing with displaced anger, then we can clarify the anger. Very often, parents are angry at the child for having the disability. Because this anger is hard to acknowledge, it is easier for them to be angry at me, because I in some sense represent the disorder. I can clarify that they actually are angry at the situation in which they find themselves. This displaced anger very often can get rechanneled into more useful places, such as working to help other parents and other children trying to live with the disability. Anger can be a very useful source of energy, especially if directed at politicians and bureaucrats who are inadequately funding programs.

There is never any loss in dealing openly and honestly with anger. It took me a long time to recognize that anger will not emerge unless there is a high degree of trust and intimacy in a relationship. Only secure people can afford to risk the loss of relationships by showing anger. Relationships are almost always strengthened after anger emerges if there is an acceptance of the feeling and a mutual willingness to explore the sources of the anger. The professional needs to be a secure person to allow client anger to emerge. If the groundwork has been laid in establishing trust, then the relationship can withstand and grow from controversy.

Guilt

I think that next to anger, guilt is the single most pervasive feeling experienced by the families of clients with disabilities. All parents, especially the mothers, feel some guilt for a child who has a congenital condition. I think guilt, in general, is more prevalent in the female population, reflecting the way that girls are acculturated in our society. They are not allowed to feel powerful; rather, they are expected to be compliant and passive. Guilt becomes a power statement: It says that I have had some negative power to influence and/or cause this bad result. One mother in a parent group once said, "I even feel guilty when it rains." My response was, "Boy, you must be feeling very powerful, too." There is also power in worry. My mother-in-law, worrier par excellence, does this all the time; the implicit statement in what she is doing is that if she worries about an event, she can control it, and thus feel some sense of power.

I have found guilt in many spouses of people with a chronic illness. For example, one guilt-ridden wife thought that her husband's Alzheimer's disease was caused by her not monitoring his nutrition carefully enough. There was also the husband who felt that he might have caused his wife's stroke by being involved in a car accident in which his wife hit her head. This was six months before the actual stroke, but when a catastrophic event happens, we always look back to find a cause and try to affix blame.

Mothers, in particular, are prone and vulnerable to guilt where children are involved. Mothers almost invariably take responsibility for causing disorders. Mothers in traditional relationships assume responsibility for the health and education of the family, and their guilt revolves around the failure to protect the family from the disorder. The causes of many congenital disorders are unknown, and parents frequently look back on the pregnancy to find a cause. This incessant search for a cause often reflects the desire to alleviate the very uncomfortable guilt feeling. Parents want to be absolved of their guilt and hope to find a cause for which they cannot be held responsible. Unfortunately, many times a cause cannot be determined. If left to their own devices, mothers will examine minutely all the details of their pregnancy and can usually locate a "cause." It is impossible to go nine months in a pregnancy without something untoward happening, and thus is born the "guilty secret." Mothers may, for example, feel that they caused the handicap by not taking their vitamins or by taking too many saunas or by smoking or drinking. Although most of these guilty secrets are unfounded and cannot stand up to rational examination, the mother often takes the blame and behaves in ways that are not productive for her or the child.

A trusting, intimate relationship between the mother and the professional must be established so that the parent feels free to discuss "this awful thing" she has done to cause her child's handicap. The nonjudgmental, unconditional regard of the humanistic-based relationship can establish the healing environment in which she will reveal the guilty secret; this is when sensitively given information can be helpful. We can bestow no greater gift than to relieve a parent of unfounded guilt.

The feeling of guilt can also stem from the client's religious feelings and experiences. For many clients and their families, the disorder becomes a reflection of their own sins. Many parents, if they can't find something in the pregnancy on which to pin the disorder, will find something in their past life to account for the disorder; even if they can't recall the sin, God must have, to have given them this child. Here again, we must be sensitive to the multicultural differences of our clients and their families.

Guilt is a difficult emotion with which to deal. The flip side of guilt is resentment, but unlike anger, resentment is seldom expressed directly; it simmers and sabotages relationships. Relationships that are built around guilt/resentment are not healthy. They usually founder and almost always fail to grow because the parties feel controlled by their guilt. There is always an external locus of control in guilt. Unfortunately, because guilt is a powerful controller of behavior, it often is used to govern children and spouses. Those families with a high degree of guilt/resentment are not healthy for children because it leads to simmering resentment. Parents who feel guilt about their child usually experience resentment as well. A child will sense the resentment and react negatively to it. There is a lot of conflict in guilt-ridden relationships. This is seldom productive conflict, though, because it is often difficult to get to the guilt issue.

Most parents are driven by their guilty feelings, and guilty parents tend to overprotect their children. Their reasoning is that "we let something bad happen to our child once and we are not about to let anything else happen." These parents do not let their child develop much autonomy or initiative. They seldom let their child out of their sight and are uncomfortable when they do. The overprotection extends to the therapy situation: The guilt-ridden parents, not very trusting of the professionals or of professional competency, question the therapist and frequently seek other opinions. It is very hard to maintain a long-term relationship with a guilt-driven parent.

Guilt feelings also lead to the superdedicated parent who reasons that "I let something bad happen to my child and now I am going to make it up to him." This parent works very hard at doing lessons with the child and attending all workshops and evening meetings. Teachers invariably exclaim,

"I wish we had more parents like them." What is not realized is the high cost that such dedication has on the family structure. The husband–wife relationship is invariably strained because so much energy is put into the parenting that very little is left for the marriage, and the child's siblings are also at risk because they receive diminished attention.

The biggest damage is probably inflicted on the superdedicated parent and on the child with the disability. Such dedication leaves these parents little or no room to develop any other aspects of their potential, and there is limited life experience outside of being parents of a child with a disability. Although these parents look very good in the preschool years when their dedication is usually reflected in high achieving youngsters, they look very bad at that point in the life cycle when their developmental task is to let go of their adolescent children and they are not able to do it. This parent wonders, "If I am not a parent of a child with a disability, who am I?" These guilt-ridden, superdedicated parents make it very hard for children to break away as they must in order to grow. All parents find late adolescence a very hard time, but if their guilt is unresolved, they find the situation almost impossible.

In counseling, the guilt issue must be dealt with in order for the family to function effectively. I tell parents that I have never yet met a hearing parent who wanted to have a deaf child or deliberately set about causing deafness in a child. When the parent actually has been guilty of some dereliction that did cause the deafness, we talk about creating an expiation contract to enable the parent to "pay back" the child or other children, without becoming a superdedicated or overprotective parent. The contract, arrived at after much discussion and thought, usually involves something like the parent's becoming an officer in a parent organization for one year. After that, the parent is to consider that he or she has paid his or her dues.

When the guilty secret is based on ignorance, such as thinking that the failure to take a vitamin pill caused the deafness, then information can help to alleviate the painful guilt feelings. When parents feel neurotic guilt built on the feelings of powerlessness and lack of control, anything we do that empowers parents will diminish the need for the guilty feelings.

In any event, a major goal of counseling should be to disengage the parent's or spouse's guilty feelings from the nonproductive behavior. People can feel guilty and still behave in a self-enhancing way. One parent said to me once, "You know, I still have all those unpleasant feelings but they don't control me anymore." She was a highly successful parent.

Feelings of Vulnerability

An existential fact of life is that we all are vulnerable. If we live long enough, something bad will happen to us, and if we don't live long enough, then something bad has already happened. To allay the anxiety caused by this fact of life, we develop a myth of invulnerability. We think bad things can't happen to us—they happen only to other people. To a large extent, we need this myth to function in our daily lives. Without it, we might never get into an airplane or drive a car; we might just spend our time cowering under the covers, and even then, we would not be safe. There is no safety in life. Nobody gets out of it alive.

When something bad does happen to us, such as having a deaf child, we feel that our cloak of invulnerability has been pierced. We realize how naked and alone we really are, and how fragile our existence is. We have lost the pseudo-comfort that the myth of invulnerability provided. This realization is scary and it may make us timid for a time. Parents undergoing a "crisis of vulnerability" seem very much like guilt-ridden, overprotective parents. A mother whose child was deafened by meningitis said,

> When I took her home from the hospital I wouldn't let her outside at all, and I wouldn't let any other children come in and play because I was afraid she might get sick again. When I finally did take her with me to the supermarket, I brought along a can of disinfectant and sprayed the shopping cart. For the first year I lived in complete terror that she might get sick again.

The anxiety generated by the awareness of vulnerability, as opposed to the anxiety that is generated from unresolved guilt feelings, can be a positive force. When we recognize our vulnerabilities, we can and very often do reorder our priorities. We can live more fully as we recognize the finiteness of our existence. The mother with the meningitic child also said:

> It made you more aware of things, more appreciative. It made me kind of stop and smell the flowers a lot more than I would before. I was always kind of rushing around and hurrying and not stopping as much as I do now. I'm just kind of enjoying everything as much as possible because you just realize, I don't know, maybe your vulnerability. Who knows what is going to happen next, so you might as well enjoy now. I used to think that that could never happen to me . . . but I don't feel that way anymore. Not in a real negative, pessimistic kind of thing, but it's life and you have no control over it, so you might as well appreciate what you have. Make the best of it.

That statement could have been written by any existential philosopher. If we allow parents to go through the grief process and we treat them with the loving respect they need, then all sorts of good things can happen to them. They can learn to take each day for the gift that it is, and although their life is not "Italy," "Holland" also has a lot to offer.

Feelings of Confusion

Almost all of our clients, as they go through the learning process, experience confusion. Confusion is a normal, healthy part of the process of learning; as we attempt to acquire new information that we do not have the experience to evaluate, and a vocabulary that is totally unfamiliar to us, we are confused. In the resolution of the confusion we learn, provided we are given time and repetition. Unfortunately, clients and their families, especially in the early stages of diagnosis, are given much more information than they can use. (See Chapter 1 for the effects of information counseling.) Professionals often use jargon and assume that after defining a term once or twice, the client has retained the meaning, which is usually not the case. We are often not aware of our jargon. Terms such as *audiogram, audiologists,* and *decibel* are rather esoteric and unfamiliar to most people. I have found, for example, that parents of deaf children take about a year to understand an audiogram despite the many tests given to their children and the many explanations given by the audiologist. (At that, they are faster than some students in my beginning audiology class.)

Professionals are not the only source of "information" to clients. One of the things that happens when someone has an apparent disability is that he or she loses anonymity. The person can hardly walk outside without other people telling their inspirational story and rendering advice. Walking with my wife in a wheelchair, for example, is an adventure. She gets "God blessed" right and left, and people offer all kinds of free advice. If we weren't pretty secure in what we know, this avalanche of well-intended advice and information would bring us to despair rather than enlightenment. Information overload can be very harmful, because the increased confusion leads to increased feelings of inadequacy and anxiety, all of which tend to reduce client self-esteem.

Professionals contribute to client confusion by providing information-based counseling when the client is not ready psychologically to receive it. For me as an insecure professional, content counseling was the prime distancing strategy. If I focused a relationship on content (which also met both the parents' and my expectations), then I could be in control and we did not need to tap into the feelings of grief and anger, with which I was very uncomfortable. This strategy severely limited the relationship, defining me as the source of knowledge, and extended the client's confusion and anxiety by providing him or her with too much gratuitous information, too early in the grief process.

As professionals, we have a responsibility to provide information. As a general rule of thumb, I do not give clients information unless they ask for it. I generally ask, "What do you need to know?" When I receive a response such as, "I don't even know enough to ask a question!" which is fairly typical in the early stages, I might respond, "It sounds like you are pretty confused." This is an invitation to talk about client feelings. I have seen professionals who are anxious to get things going tell parents who are too confused to ask questions, "Here are some things I think you need to know." This response must be resisted at all costs because it takes away client power and gives the professional too much responsibility. The content questions will emerge as the clients become more comfortable with their new status and are moved a bit further along in the grief process. If we facilitate the process by empathetic listening, the content will emerge.

When clients ask specific content questions, I answer them. I like to think that my answers are free of opinion, but I, like most professionals in the field, have strong opinions. The best I can do is to identify them as opinions when talking with the parents. There is a need and a place for content, even in the early stages of relationships; it fulfills an implicit contract between professionals and their clients. I feel that in the initial stages, the information functions more to establish credibility than to alleviate ignorance. This must occur in order for us to be truly helpful, but we also must remain sensitive to the relationship as it is being established.

These feelings—grief, anxiety, inadequacy, anger, guilt, vulnerability, and confusion—are turbulent and chaotic feelings that clients and their families experience when they encounter a disability in themselves or a family member. These people are emotionally upset, and very appropriately so. As was said at the outset of this chapter, feelings are neither good nor bad, and it is not our responsibility to make our clients feel better. We can, by our calm acceptance of their feelings and our willingness to allow affect to be part of the client–professional relationship, prevent the development of secondary negative feelings. We can, for example, help to prevent clients from feeling guilty about their guilt feelings. When we do this, their coping process can begin. With our sensitive appreciation of the grief process, the clients' chaotic feelings can be transformed into positive behavior. Thus, the grief can become a sadness that enables the clients to appreciate what they have, the anger can become the energy to make change, the guilt can become the commitment, the recognition of vulnerability can become the means by which clients reorder priorities, and the resolution of confusion can become the motivation for learning.

The Professional's Feelings

The feelings described in this chapter in relation to clients also characterize the professional's reactions. Nothing is abnormal or unhealthy about any of the feelings described. Under the skin we are all brothers and sisters. Audiologists, for example, often feel overwhelmed by and inadequate to cope with the responsibility of determining a child's hearing loss and of properly counseling the family. This is especially true of the beginning audiologist, who is still developing good test techniques and learning appropriate counseling strategies. Even veteran audiologists experience an anxiety almost akin to panic when presented with a child who promises to be difficult to test and a family that appears hard to counsel. Has any professional not felt the fear of that icy finger of failure? The anxiety becomes the spur for continued professional improvement.

Professionals also experience anger. They feel anger at parents for not following through on a recommended course of action; they feel rage, frustration, and sometimes despair when they can't make things better for the child or family with whom they are involved. They may feel intense anger at other professionals who insensitively or inappropriately treat the families: the pediatricians who fail to refer or the classroom teachers who don't understand the child's language difficulty. This anger provides the energy that can be used to educate other professionals and make programmatic changes. If repressed, it lends itself to depression and burnout.

Guilt is also a part of the professional's experience. I know of no responsible and competent speech and hearing professional who suffers no regrets about the handling of past cases. Mistakes—an inevitable part of the experience of all professionals—are our "nuggets of gold." They indicate to us what we need to learn next. All responsible professionals should be operating on their "fringes of incompetence." They should be taking risks and occasionally making mistakes, or they are not growing. Many speech and hearing professionals are needlessly burdened by the guilt associated with their errors. Fortunately, we are not brain surgeons. Almost all my clients have survived my mistakes quite well. Some have even flourished; so have I.

Those of us who work clinically, especially in hospital settings, are constantly confronted with people who have severe disorders. We are not given the luxury that most people have of retaining our myth of invulnerability. Daily we meet people like us who are in deep pain and we often say, "There but for the grace of God go I." The recognition of our personal vulnerability can lead to our being very caring, thoughtful clinicians, and it can spill over into our personal lives where we can reorder our priorities, much as our clients do when they realize what is really important in life.

Frequently when the feelings surrounding communication disorders are described, the negative and painful emotions are emphasized, while the positive feelings and experiences are seldom discussed. Often overlooked are the marvelous opportunities for joy and growth. Many parents come through the experience of having a hearing-impaired child with a clearer sense of themselves and of their priorities than they had before their child was diagnosed. Many parents discover that their child's disorder has given their life meaning and direction. The joy stems from actively participating in their child's growth; they take nothing for granted. When their child reaches a milestone, they rejoice in the knowledge that they helped in the accomplishment. I am always reminded of the Bertrand Russell quote, "To be without some of the things you want is an indispensable part of happiness."

The speech and hearing professional also experiences joy in working with the families of clients. In the initial stages of diagnosis, everything appears bleak and hopeless to the families, and the speech pathologist or audiologist often becomes their lifeline. My most meaningful clinical experiences have been in the intimate relationships that I have had with parents of newly diagnosed hearing-impaired children. It is very gratifying to witness and participate actively in the process by which people grow and fulfill their potential. I often tell parents that I will share some of their pain if they will share some of their joy with me as well.

Training Students for Parent Programs

If there is going to be any meaningful change in the current parent–professional relationship, it will have to occur at the professional training level. Too many young clinicians leave their training programs with minimal or very inadequate experience in relating to parents. I suspect that part of the problem lies in the lack of practice in parent training of the supervisors and academic teachers in their training programs. The new ASHA regulations allow 25 clock hours of student activity with parents to be counted toward the 375 hours needed for certification. Cartwright and Ruscello (1979) suggested that 10% of the total student contact hours with parents be allowed to count for certification, which seems quite reasonable to me.

On a national level, we also need to promote continuing education workshops specifically geared toward professionals in academic programs on the utilization of parents and the training of students in parent involvement. We need to increase the number and quality of our parent involvement programs throughout the nation. Only half of all approved clinics have a parent involvement program (Cartwright & Ruscello, 1979). This figure seems inadequate to me, especially since nearly 90% of all programs report that parent involvement is very important. We should also be very concerned about the quality of the parent programming. There are too many professional-centered parent programs (i.e., programs in which the professional has the control and uses the educational program to promote a particular point of view) in which the personal growth of the parents is minimal. A good parent program has to be designed with the parent in mind. If we try to append a parent program onto an existing child-centered program, we are doomed to failure. The program rapidly becomes the PTA model of parent involvement, which usually entails hurried parent conferences and lectures in which parents are talked at rather than listened to. In good programming, the parent is the primary target.

Good parent programs have a snowball effect. They produce self-confident, positively assertive parents who will work as equals with other professionals. These parents, in effect, become trainers of all professionals. They open the eyes of professionals to the potential of parent involvement. The reasonably self-confident professional finds it a relief to have a parent as a co-worker.

If parent–professional relationships are to improve, they have to be freed from a problem-centered orientation. Much of the contact between parent and professional occurs only when there is a specific problem. It is very hard to have a productive relationship when it is always problem centered. I give my aural rehabilitation class a role-playing situation in which a teacher of deaf students calls a parent to school to tell the parent that his or her child is "an oral failure" and should be put in a total communication program. The problem is set up to be adversarial in that the parent is strongly committed to an oral education. The situation usually ends up in disaster, in part because if this is the first parent–professional meeting (as generally happens), it is already too late. Time has not been spent in developing the necessary trust, autonomy, and initiative before they can deal with such a loaded topic as changing the mode of communication for the child.

Some of my students solve this problem well. They recognize that the person with the problem is the teacher, not the parent or the child. When the teacher can convey to the parent that the teacher has a problem and can enlist the parent's help, then the relationship does not become adversarial. Both parent and teacher can embark together on a quest to find the best way of educating the child. It is also agreed by the class after the role-playing activity that the teacher should have seen the parents outside of the school and established and worked on their relationship before any problems occurred.

Parents and professionals in speech–language pathology are natural allies. They both want in the most ardent terms the same thing: a child with better communicating skills. Murphy (1981), in an almost lyrically written and lovely book on parents, *Special Children, Special Parents,* wrote, "Parents and workers are sculptors helping to shape what a child may become. There is a place for all—a place to be, to become something more than they now are, a place to learn, to dance, to sing" (p. ix).

The Coping Process

Recently in my research on chronic illness, I came across a coping process model that I have found very helpful in many of my clinical interactions. Again, the model is useful only as a guide, and the stages are not firmly fixed points as in climbing a mountain—once gained never lost—but rather a fluid series of points in which even successfully coping individuals return to earlier stages. Matson and Brooks (1977), in their interviews with patients who had multiple sclerosis, found four stages to the coping process: denial, resistance, affirmation, and integration.

Let us look at these stages in relation to communication disorders.

Denial

Probably no single factor impairs client–professional relationships as much as the denial mechanism. Denial must be seen by the professional for what it is, namely, a coping strategy based on feelings of inadequacy. When a person is in denial, there is no psychological "owning" of the problem. The person may admit that the problem exists, but emotionally, he or she is not engaged. Denial is a very normal, very human reaction that occurs in all of us.

When I am driving my car, for example, and the engine begins to sound strange, I respond by turning on the radio. If the engine noises get louder, I increase the volume. Although I know cognitively that turning on the radio is not going to solve my problem, at that time, psychologically, it is the only thing I can do. In short, I try to deny the existence of the problem, hoping that it will go away by itself. My need to adopt the radio strategy is based on my lack of confidence in my ability to repair engines. I feel totally inadequate around mechanical things, certainly anything as complicated as a car engine. If you were to admonish me about how silly I am to respond by turning on the radio, I would grin sheepishly and agree with you. At this point I use a passive–aggressive strategy that I learned as a child in how to deal with authority figures—that is, I agree with you and proceed to do what I was doing when you are not around. Unless I am given other ways of coping and gain some confidence in myself, I cannot afford to give up denial. If, for example, I successfully completed a course in engine maintenance with your help, then I might hear the slightest noise and pull the car to the side of the road because I feel I have some chance of solving the problem and I would therefore cope with the crisis in a more responsible way than by denying its existence.

Parents of a child with a disability begin to experience feelings of denial any time there is a new demand on parental resources, requiring that they be wise or strong. The most obvious time is at diagnosis: Often the delay in getting a child diagnosed is because the parents cannot admit to themselves that something may be wrong. Others in the parents' environment also practice denial, especially grandparents, and sometimes professionals such as the family pediatrician.

Denial persists even when the parents freely acknowledge that they have a child with a disability. In coping with deafness, denial occurs around anything that objectifies the deafness. The hearing aid, for example, becomes a powerful reminder of deafness. Parents may hate to see it on their child even though they know it helps. When they take pictures of the child, they remove the hearing aid. This, by the way, becomes a good measure of where the parents are on the coping model. Parents who are in the affirmation or integration stage insist that the hearing aid be worn, whereas those who are in the denial or resistance stage remove it for pictures. If the parents are in a total communication program, their denial can become focused on the signing; thus we have parents who never attend class or, when they do, cannot seem to learn how to sign.

The child-centered professional views parental denial as an impediment to the child's progress and gets angry at the parents. The professional who is direct about the anger gives the parents an admonitory lecture about how important it is for the child to wear the aid or how necessary it is for the parents to attend signing class. The parents agree with the professional; they knew how important it was before the professional told them, but because they have no other coping strategy—much as I didn't with my car—they fall back on denial. After an initial period of attendance at classes or increased hearing-aid use, they often revert to denial, which provokes another round of professional ire. If not stopped, this negative parent–professional interaction can escalate to the point where there is no communication between parent and professional, to the detriment of the child.

The professional must learn to recognize the denial as a plea for help, and not as a dereliction of duty on the parents' part. No parents, at least those whom I have met, want to do badly by their child, but their many fears get in the way of their operating constructively. The basis of denial is fear and ignorance abetted by low self-esteem. People cannot be urged out of denial. They give it up when they feel confident that they can be more successful with some other strategy. In general, it is best not to undermine the denial mechanism directly unless one has something better to offer in its stead. Giving up denial—the only way the clients feel that they can currently cope with the situation—with nothing to replace it would be overwhelming. The parents feel as if their psychological survival depends on denial, and in some respects it does. Denial is not given up easily. By listening and by indirect teaching, which does not diminish clients' feelings of competency, counselors can teach clients more fruitful coping strategies than denial.

If the professional is focused on the child and is anxious about the child's welfare, parental denial might provoke an adversarial relationship between the professional and the parents that can destroy any productive counseling relationship. Professionals often try to "save" the child from the parents. Short of removing the child from the home, this cannot be done. Children cannot be saved from their parents; all of us, in some sense, are victims of our parents' failings. The professional must not let parental denial impair the development of a healthy relationship. I don't think any successful counseling can take place unless the professional has some understanding of the denial mechanism.

The identification of behavior as denial can be very tricky. It is not always clear when the clients are denying or when there is a legitimate difference of opinion between the client and the professional. Labeling can be used to try to substitute professional "truth" for parental "truth"—and room must be allowed for a difference of opinion.

One person's denial may be another person's optimism. Frequently, when the professional has a very pessimistic prognosis for a child, the parent keeps saying, "He will make it." Children have a way of meeting expectations, and when the expectations are negative, children seldom perform well. I have often seen the parents proved right; there is never any need to diminish parental optimism as long as their behavior is consistent with accepted management practices. The optimism frequently gets translated into hope, and many parents have the "maybe someday they will find a cure" dream. This dream, which enables them to work vigorously in the present and sustains them when they despair, should never be doused by the professional. There is probably no crueler act than to deprive the parents of this dream.

There is also much that is positive about denial. In 1962, the U.S. government declared Spanish–American War veterans, of which there were only several hundred in the United States, totally disabled. This declaration, which entitled them to receive full benefits at the Veterans' Administration, occasioned the launching of a large-scale study of the aged male. These men were in their 80s at the time, and the study involved gathering data on all aspects of their lives. I was involved in studying their hearing. As part of the examination, I interviewed them about how well they thought they could hear. This part of the research protocol became meaningless, as every one of them felt he could hear fine, despite the fact that in many instances I had to shout to be heard. I spoke to the project psychologist about this phenomenon, and he said it was pervasive throughout the study. These men persistently denied any infirmity, and he concluded—only partially tongue in cheek—that perhaps one of the major secrets of living to a ripe old age is to assiduously practice denial.

Resistance

Denial blends into resistance and at times is indistinguishable from it. In the resistance stage, the client and the family say, "We have a problem here but we are going to be a special case. We will somehow prevail over the disorder." Parents of a deaf child, for instance, say, "I know he is deaf but he is going to be a super deaf person. He will have normal speech, be a marvelous lipreader, and have an amazing job that few people will ever expect a deaf person to have." My wife, shortly after being diagnosed as having multiple sclerosis, ran a 10-k race as though to defiantly say, "Being a cripple won't happen to me." As I watched her stagger across the finish line, I was filled with both admiration and anxiety for her. That was the last race she ever ran.

Resistance differs from denial in that the persons acknowledge to themselves that they have a problem and they work very hard to defeat it. In resistance, there is almost always a private pledge to conquer the disorder, and a rejection of help from any organizations that deal with the disorder. During the resistance stage, clients are unwilling to join any support groups or receive help in the form of meeting with peer counselors. They are in effect "closet" disabled. In the early stages of diagnosis, my wife and I did not, for example, want to meet anyone who had multiple sclerosis, and I still find it very hard if not impossible to go to meetings where there are adults who are severely disabled by the condition. I just don't want to be reminded of my potential future. (My wife is much better at this than I am.)

In resistance, a great deal of energy is directed almost frantically and secretly at proving that the professionals were "wrong." Both denial and resistance are used to forestall or minimize the pain of the grief process. In denial, one says, "I don't really have this problem." In resistance, the person says, "I will lick this problem."

The difficulty for clients and their families comes about when they realize that they have a disorder that they cannot defeat. For parents of a deaf child, this sometimes happens as late as the child's adolescence, when they realize that he or she is not going to be the super deaf adult that they had expected; another dream dies and the grief process starts anew.

Clients often need to hit an emotional bottom in order to move on with the coping process. They need to see for themselves that denial does not work and that frantic resistance is not productive before they can mourn deeply their loss and move into the affirmation stage. To move to that stage, they need to have some confidence in their own ability to cope with the disorder in a proactive manner.

Affirmation

In the affirmation stage, the loss is acknowledged both to self and to the world at large. Affirmation is a statement that "I am now a different person and our family is also different." During this stage of coping, the family is consumed by the disorder. Energy is devoted toward ameliorating the effects of the disorder. In this stage, families become very active in organizations designed to educate the members and the public at large. One such group, SHHH (Self Help for the Hard of Hearing), is designed as a support/educational group for the hard-of-hearing. In groups such as SHHH, members get an opportunity to establish their new identity as "hard-of-hearing persons"; they have come out of the disability closet. The new identity may be taken on tentatively or proudly (as we have seen in the deaf community), but it is a public acknowledgment of the new identity. In this stage, an intense desire to help others arises. One parent of a deaf child said, "When you first find out your child is deaf, you feel badly for yourself. After a while you feel badly for your child. Now I feel badly for all deaf children." This movement outside of one's own pain is very healthy and marks the transition into integration.

Integration

Integration (also known as acceptance) is characterized by getting the disorder into a life perspective. The client and family learn to live with the disorder and to spend time and energy on other matters. The client is able to say, "I am more than a walking hearing disorder; I am a person who does not hear well, but many other aspects of my life need to be developed." In the integration/acceptance stage, although there is still pain for the loss, and at times grief, the changes caused by the disorder are integrated into a new lifestyle with different values. The affirmation and acceptance stages are reached when the individual realizes that "beating" the disorder is not always a matter of reaching normalcy, but rather the ability to live life to the fullest in the face of the disorder.

Individuals vary as to the degree and speed with which they can get to integration. Some families seem forever stuck in denial, which seems to them to be the only possible coping strategy; they are paralyzed in their fear. Others move through the process very rapidly, seeming to skip stages. The key is the self-confidence of the families. When they feel secure in their abilities to cope, it becomes easier to assume the psychological risk of giving up the pseudo-comfort of denial and resistance to assume the responsibilities demanded by the affirmation and integration stages of the coping process. Let us look now specifically at coping.

Coping

My dictionary defines *coping* as "contending successfully with." All coping involves a stressful interaction between a person and the environment.

Coping is any response to a difficult life situation that avoids or prevents distress. Successful coping always involves the possibility of growth and always demands change. It is the people who are uncomfortable who will grow because they are forced to derive a new set of responses to contend with a changing set of either internal or external demands. We tend to give to life what life demands of us, and when we are stressed by an external force, we must find within us the strength and develop within us the resources to cope successfully. Coping is a dynamic process; it is not a stage finally won and held forever. At times it is a moment-to-moment proposition.

Pearlin and Schooler (1978), in a definitive article on coping, outlined four strategies that individuals use to cope with very difficult situations: flight, modification, reframing, and stress reduction.

Flight

The first and perhaps primary coping strategy is flight. Each person when confronted with a difficult and potentially stressful situation must decide whether to fight or take flight. In some situations in life, a person feels ill-equipped to survive and that his or her own personal or psychological survival depends on removal from the situation. This may not be the reality of the situation, but as long as people feel that they cannot cope successfully, then flight will occur. It is the person's perception of events that is critical.

Many divorces occur in families with children with disabilities and estrangements in families with adults with disabilities. Sometimes an adult child leaves a parent to struggle alone with a spouse with a disability. As a coping strategy, flight always leaves the person vulnerable to guilt and loss of self-esteem. In addition to the actual flight, as in a divorce, there is the psychological flight that occurs very frequently in parents and spouses of family members with disabilities. The psychological flight often takes the form of a fantasy about the death of the child or spouse. This is a deep-seated "wish" that is difficult for many parents or spouses to admit because they feel enormously guilty about having these feelings. When they do admit these fantasies to a professional, there usually is a high degree of trust in the relationship and they expect the professional to accept their statement at face value. It is critical that the professional accepts this admission in a matter-of-fact manner. These feelings are very common. I often tell parents and spouses that I don't think they are wishing their child or spouse dead, but that they are wishing this situation, which is so stressful to them, would go away.

Death fantasies may be helpful in preparing for the actual death of a spouse. This anticipatory mourning is seen frequently in spouses of clients with aphasia and in families in which someone has traumatic head injuries. Anticipatory mourning, which helps the person make the adjustment to living without the person with a disability, is part of the psychologically protective transition process that eases the way into an anticipated new status. The person is trying on the new role, which is very helpful, although it generally causes the person to feel a great deal of guilt. Professionals must never judge these fantasies, which almost always serve a useful psychological function as long as they remain fantasies.

Modification

If a person decides to stay with the family member with a disability, then the next strategy employed is to modify the situation. Stress can be reduced by direct intervention that reduces or modifies the disability. The client who gets a hearing aid and the patient with aphasia who gets a wheelchair and language therapy may reduce the stress caused by their losses. All therapy administered by a speech and hearing clinician is designed to reduce stress and help clients and their families cope better with communication situations.

Unfortunately, in our field there are many situations in which the stress of a disorder can be modified but not eliminated. For example, even with the best amplification, many clients will still have a significant hearing loss. We must help these clients to accept their limitations and to recognize that they cannot modify their environment any further. The trick in trying to modify the stressful situation is to know what can be modified and do it, and then learn to accept what cannot be changed—not always easy to do.

Reframing

Because the cognitive process always determines the emotional intensity of any event, for those elements of a situation that cannot be modified, stress can be reduced by changing the way a person views the situation. This is known as *reframing* or cognitively neutralizing the stressor. The most commonly used cognitive neutralizer is the phrase, "It could be worse," whereupon parents or spouses proceed to mention someone, someplace who is in more difficulty than they are. This is known as a positive comparison. The problem with using positive comparisons as a reframing strategy is that there are still times when the client or the family member feels upset about the disability. When this happens, they usually feel guilty because they feel they have forfeited their right to grieve. My wife's response to, "It could be worse," is to say, "Yes and it could be better, too!"

Using positive comparisons often buys some short-term relief, but the disability will always intrude, and the effectiveness of looking for someone worse off begins to fade quickly. There are other more fruitful ways of reframing, which are discussed in Chapter 6.

Stress Reduction

The fourth strategy is to deal directly with the stress. No matter how successful modification and reframing might be, many clients will still experience stress with which they must learn to live. Each individual must find his or her own individual stress reducers, and what is effective for one person may not work for another. In my interviews with the spouses of patients with chronic illness, I found that exercise and work are almost universal stress reducers. Exercise is effective in part because it is a time-out experience that gets the well spouse away from confronting the spouse with a disability. It also is an emotionally calming activity. Especially repetitive exercise, such as jogging, swimming, or bicycling, seems to put the mind into a meditative state. Work serves as a distraction. Well spouses can immerse themselves in problems that have solutions and are controllable. They also are in contact with other adults with whom they can talk and think about something other than their spouses. In fact, one of my definitions of a "shadow spouse" is someone who looks forward to going to work and dreads coming home.

When speech and hearing professionals encounter clients, the traumatic events have already happened, and the grief and coping processes are already under way. By virtue of the way we interact with clients and their families, we can facilitate or retard the coping process. This is especially true at the diagnostic evaluation, which is usually close to the time of the catastrophic event, when clients' feelings are very fluid and apparent; because the impact of the disorder has not settled in yet, we can alter very dramatically the course of the coping and the habilitation of the client.

5

Counseling and
the Diagnostic Process

The diagnostic interaction is critical for determining the future course of the client–professional relationship. It is the first step on a long journey for many clients, and it is an imprinting process that sets up in the client's mind future expectations of professional behavior. If the initial client–professional interaction has a feeling component and if clients are empowered at the outset, then they will expect and perhaps demand empowerment and affect in future contacts with professionals. Unfortunately, because of the prevalence of the medical model, the professional's role is usually restricted to providing information and prescribing what the client should do. In this model, the client is encouraged to become a passive participant in the habilitation program by simply "following the doctor's orders."

Institution-Centered Diagnosis

In the medical model, a careful case history is obtained and tests are given. If a child is being tested, he or she is separated from the parents while the professional administers the tests. (If the parent is allowed to be present, it is usually as a very passive observer.) After the testing, the professional "counsels" the parents by giving the results of the tests and recommending what the parents should do next. As a beginning audiologist, I found the medical model very helpful. I soon developed some set speeches that I could give at the end of testing a child. They were like "tapes" I could plug in to describe how hearing aids worked, explain audiograms, and, for parents of newly diagnosed deaf children, provide a list of schools for the deaf in the area and describe the various educational methodologies utilized in the schools. On the surface, the medical model seems very efficient. Because I could control the interaction time, I could block out a prescribed time and see the maximum number of cases in a given day. I could fit each speech into a 10- or 15-minute period and then send the parents on their way, feeling that I had fulfilled my clinical obligation, and perhaps as importantly, I could see my next patient on time. I also succeeded in limiting the affective exchange so that I did not have to deal with feelings, about which I felt very insecure. After a while I stopped "seeing" patients; the visits simply became very routine and mechanical for me.

A variation of the individual medical model is the diagnosis-by-committee process, which on the surface is even more efficient. Many hospitals and educational programs operate this way when they have, for example, an individual educational plan (IEP). In this model, the child is tested by an array of professionals, usually on the same day, but sometimes spread over two or three days. The parents are then invited to a conference at which each professional delivers his or her report. Professionals in these meetings seldom talk directly to the parents: They are so busy trying to impress everyone else with their competency that they are speaking to impress rather then express; jargon abounds. Parents are glassy-eyed and generally traumatized by the whole experience. Imagine the experience from the parents' perspective of having a group of "experts" sitting around a table telling you what is wrong with your child. It has to be a nightmare!

Currently at Emerson College, research is under way in which parents who have undergone the diagnosis-by-committee process are interviewed. They report that they retained almost none of the material presented to them. They report feeling very scared and very numb. We have yet to find any parents who liked or appreciated the experience. At best, they found it helpful "because they didn't have to make so many trips to the hospital." All found it psychologically painful.

My personal opinion is that diagnosis by committee should be banned by the Geneva Convention as cruel and unusual punishment. It is utilized because it seems efficient to be able in one fell swoop to have the complete diagnosis. The efficiency is only illusory. Diagnosis by committee is convenient for the institution or the professionals; it is not efficient when one examines its effects on the families. Instead of retaining much of what is said, they remember unimportant details such as the color of the doctor's tie or the kind of glasses he or she wore. They always remember the date vividly, and can describe the trip to the hospital in explicit detail, but they usually fail to retain any of the important information (Martin et al., 1990).

The value of any diagnostic process can only be as good as the counseling techniques and procedures employed. Of what use is it to have highly accurate tests and highly "efficient" procedures if you cannot communicate them effectively to the clients? The data we have indicate that the medical model is not an effective tool whether it be by committee or by individuals. The research cited in Chapter 1 (Lerner, 1988; Martin et al., 1987; Williams & Derbyshire, 1982) shows how little parents retain of the information provided and how little they trust the audiologist. There are much better ways to conduct a diagnostic examination, which, although it may involve more time in the initial stages, will be much more efficient in the long term. The recommended approach is client centered, as opposed to the institution-centered approach of the medical model.

Client-Centered Diagnosis

For a good diagnostic examination, it is important that the professional understand and have some empathy for the client's history. When clients are first seen in the clinic, they bring with them a long history of their personal struggles with the realization that something is wrong. For example, a scenario for the parents of a congenitally deaf child might be something like this: One parent, usually the mother, becomes aware that something is wrong with the child. The first fear that parents frequently have when they suspect something is wrong is that their child might be mentally retarded. (Retardation is generally what parents fear the most and are most likely to fixate on.) When the mother begins to localize problems to the hearing, she confides her fears to the father, who responds by denying it, reassuring his wife and himself that nothing is wrong with their baby. At this point, each parent embarks on a surreptitious program of testing the child's hearing without confiding their fears to each other. Now the parents are on an emotional roller coaster; they are elated when they get a response or a pseudo-response, and crushed when the child fails to respond. They often elicit pseudo-responses, for example, by banging pans together behind the child's back (which creates a pressure wave that the child feels or casts a shadow on the wall that is evident within the child's peripheral vision) or by making a sound loud enough that the child responds legitimately even though there is a substantial hearing loss.

The denial mechanism is activated very early during this self-diagnosis process so that parents can find many reasons as to why the child does not respond. (This is equally true for any insidious neurological disease. My wife and I, for example, spent a great deal of time explaining away her vague neurological symptoms; one becomes an expert at finding benign reasons for frighteningly deviant behavior.) This period of uncertainty is very painful as the individuals vacillate between the peaks of relief and the valleys of fear and anxiety. Finally, the denial mechanism, battered by the assault of accumulated data, gives way, and with a great deal of trepidation the families approach a professional for a diagnosis of the disorder. At this point, the parents have generally agreed that something is wrong; they sustain themselves with the thought that medical science will be able to cure the disorder. They think that if their child is deaf, an operation or a device will enable the child to hear again. (My wife and I hoped that the neurologist would be able to recommend a drug or a course of action that would cure the disorder or at least prevent further decline in her functioning. I remember also hoping that he would simply attribute her symptoms to increasing age.) All clients come to the diagnostic situation with the knowledge that there is something wrong but also with some sustaining hope. It is the dashing of this hope that is so painful and that initiates the grief reaction.

Clients are always very anxious when they arrive at the clinic. They do not know what to expect; they are hoping against hope that they are wrong. They have composed a story detailing their experiences to date and they need to be allowed a chance to tell it to someone who will listen to them. That is why it is essential that they be given a chance to tell their story. A question such as, "Can you tell me what brought you here?" will generally elicit the story.

Client-centered counseling in the diagnostic process begins at the moment of the initial contact with the family and is continuous throughout the relationship. What needs to be established at the outset is the major concern of the parents and their expectations of the professional. Typically parents express some concern about the child's hearing or speech (although one can get very surprising answers to the question, "What concerns you most about your child?"). I don't try at this point to get a case history from the parents; I simply let them tell me anything that they think is important. Later I will get to the more specific details.

After the parents have shared their concerns and told their story, I enlist them as co-workers. I say something to them like, "I may be an expert on the testing of hearing, but you are certainly an expert on this child; I need your help."

This remark about needing help is not a ploy to get parents involved but is very much the truth. Parents have a great deal of information about the child that we can utilize in the diagnostic process. Parents can come to the testing with most of the information in hand. Dale (1991) found that parent's self-report of vocabulary and syntax of two-year-old children correlated .79 with the standardized tests administered to the children. He strongly recommended that parents' self-report be utilized in speech and language evaluations because they are

1. More representative of infant and toddler language than laboratory samples.

2. Cost-effective for a rapid general evaluation of child language.

3. Helpful in selecting assessment procedures for more in-depth analyses, if they are used before the child is seen.

4. Useful for monitoring changes that may result from intervention.

But above all else, the self-report, which enlists the parents as codiagnosticians, begins the process of empowering the parents. When I am conducting the audiological examination I also bring in any other family members who have accompanied the parents, including grandparents and siblings. If it gets too chaotic, I may ask the other family members to leave, but often they are very helpful, especially an older sibling whom I generally use to condition the child being diagnosed. I proceed to start testing the child, usually giving one parent the audiogram to fill out. In this way the information that they need is being incorporated into what they are doing and seeing. The audiogram becomes much more meaningful to them because they are using it. When I am testing an adult, I usually have a family member in the test module with me, filling in the audiogram and scoring the discrimination tests. At the time of making the appointment for the examination, it is strongly suggested that the adult with a hearing impairment be accompanied by a family member.

When a sound comes on, I describe how loud the test sound is in terms of decibels and in terms of environmental stimuli (e.g., "This sound is about as loud as people talk"). Then I ask the parents whether they thought their child heard the sound. Depending on the age of the child, we might use visual reinforcement audiometry, where a light is paired with a sound, or play audiometry, where the child is conditioned to respond to a particular sound, for example, by placing a block in a toy mailbox. If the parents and I disagree, I present the sound again until we have some agreement. At the end of the testing, I ask the parents what they think about their child's hearing and we decide whether the child has a hearing loss. If we cannot agree, we continue testing, or if the child is not cooperative, we schedule another appointment with the Scotch verdict of "not proven." I never overrule the parents' opinion. Although I might hold to my opinion that the child does have a hearing loss, I never impose it on the parents; they would lose too much power if I did this and would not be fully invested in the child's habilitation program.

Parents have recounted to me years later their feelings during this kind of testing process. They frequently report how painful it was to sit in the room and hear those loud sounds while their child showed no response. This procedure diminishes the denial mechanism because the parents actually witness the hearing impairment. There is no way out for them because the testing procedure is modified according to their perceptions, and they are the ones who actually do the diagnosis.

Clinical procedures that separate the families from the testing process frequently increase denial because the parents can fantasize about the testing (i.e., to think that maybe the machine was broken or tracings were switched or . . . or . . .). Although procedures that separate the parents might be more clinically accurate in detecting and determining the hearing loss because there are no distractions for the audiologist, they are worthless if the parents cannot or will not accept the results. Parents have a need to "view the body." There is tremendous folk wisdom in the traditional funeral ritual when people go to the funeral parlor and view a body in the open casket, and then accompany the hearse to the cemetery and watch the casket lowered into the open grave. At first this might seem cruel, but it is psychologically very sound because it diminishes the denial reaction and allows the grief process to begin. The needed restructuring of one's life because of the loss can then begin. Among the more psychologically disabled people in our society are the families of Vietnam War veterans who are still missing in action. These families cannot commit fully to a new life because they have not participated in a funeral. There is always a part of them that expects their loved ones to return, and they can imagine all sorts of scenarios in which they still might be alive. Denial in this case forestalls grief and delays or diminishes the necessary restructuring.

Active parental involvement in the diagnostic process not only diminishes the denial mechanism, but also strengthens the bond between the audiologist and the parents. Parents have reported to me how glad they were that I was there helping them through the painful process. I was seen as an ally rather than as an adversary. Audiologists who deliver the word to parents in the waiting room that their child is deaf, no matter how nicely they do it, are often received with hostility.

Another benefit of having the parents as codiagnosticians is that they are also being educated about the audiological process. The information is gradually delivered to them, and because they are participating, it is retained much more readily than when a professional delivers a "taped" speech at the end of the testing to parents who have been sitting in the waiting room. Participating parents not only understand audiograms better, but they also obtain an idea of what this child can and cannot hear in the home environment, information that becomes very useful for them in the habilitation process. Participating in this way is especially helpful for the families of adults because it lets them see the extent of the disability and enables them to effectively participate in the habilitation process.

If, after completing the testing, we decide that the child is hearing impaired, I do not supply gratuitous information. Although I know that parents "need" a lot more information to effectively manage their child's habilitation than I give on that first session, I also know that at this point I can't overwhelm them with information. At this time I ask the parents, "What do you need to know now?" and I allow them to guide their own learning experience. I usually get a few desultory questions, which I answer simply because I know that the parents are in a state of shock. Parents have told me that after the definitive diagnosis, all they wanted to do was go someplace and cry. This reaction is more from grief than from the diagnosis of deafness. Sometimes the parents actually respond to the diagnosis with relief, first because it is deafness and not retardation, of which they were mortally afraid, and second because somebody finally believed them and gave a name to the deviant behaviors of their child. With a name for the disorder, people sometimes think there is a way of controlling it. It is the information that there is no cure for the deafness that begins the grief process.

I have found over the years that one cannot go any faster with a child than the parents are willing or able to go. Audiologists limit truly effective case management when they become overwhelmed by their own anxiety to get the habilitation process moving. They then try to bypass the parental grief reaction by taking very active management of the case, leading invariably to passive, dependent parents and to ineffective long-term management of the child. I feel very strongly that if we pay careful attention to the parents during the diagnostic process by taking time for them and giving them space to grieve, then the child will do well in the long term. This may require the audiologist to let time elapse between the diagnosis and the initiation of habilitation procedures. It is difficult for most audiologists, however, to see a child needing service and not getting it immediately.

Recently I came across a poem written by a professional and a parent that captures the essence of the interpersonal, affective dimension of the diagnostic process. The poem, reprinted with permission, is as follows:

Advice to Professionals
Who Must
Conference Cases

Before the case conference,
I would look at my almost five-year-old son
And see a golden hair boy
Who giggled at his new baby sister's attempt to clap her hands,
Who charmed adults by his spontaneous hugs and hello's,
Who captured his parents with his rapture with music and
his care for white haired people who walked a walk
a bit slower than younger folks,
Who often became a legend in places visited because of his
exquisite ability to befriend a few special souls,
Who often wanted to play "peace marches,"
And who, at the age of four,
went to the Detroit Public Library
requesting a book on Martin Luther King.

After the case conference,
I looked at my almost five-year-old son.
He seemed to have lost his golden hair.
I saw only words plastered on his face.
Words that drowned us in fear and revolting nausea.

Words like:
Primary expressive speech and language disorder
severe visual motor delay
sensory integration dysfunction
fine and gross motor delay
developmental dyspraxia and
RITALIN now.

I want my son back. That's all
I want him back now. Then I'll get on with my life.
If you could feel the depth of this wrenching pain.
If you could see the depth of our sadness
then you would be moved to return
our almost five-year-old son
who sparkles in the sunlight
despite
his faulty neurons.

Please give me back my son
undamaged and
untouched by your labels, test results,
descriptions and categories

If you can't
If you truly cannot give us back our son

Then
Just be with us quietly,
gently,
and compassionately as we feel.

Just sit patiently
and attentively as
we grieve and feel powerless.

Sit with us and create a stillness known only in small, empty
chapels at sundown.
Be there
With us as our witness and
as our friend.

Please do not give us
advice,
suggestions,

comparisons or
another appointment. (That's for later.)

We want only
a quiet shoulder
upon which to rest our too-heavy heads.

If you can't give us back our sweet dream
then
comfort us through this nightmare.

Hold us.
rock us
until morning light creeps in.

Then we will rise
and begin the work of a new day.

Janice Fialka
Parent, MSW, ACSW

The second question I ask parents when we emerge from the test booth is, "Can you share with me how you are feeling?" This is an invitation to talk about affect. I sometimes give parents a bit of help by saying, "Some parents at this time feel like they have been hit by a truck," or maybe, "Some parents feel like they are walking through someone else's nightmare." Occasionally, parents begin to cry and I stay with them. My own experience has led me to believe that the parents who cry most at the initial diagnostic session do better than those parents who seem to accept the diagnosis stoically. The "criers" are usually not very adept at using denial, and they are realizing the extent of the disability rather quickly. After the initial falling apart, they usually recover quite well and get readily to work. The "stoics" very often are buttressed by denial and sometimes never make it out of denial to work effectively with their child.

A frequent mistake made by audiologists with parents of a child who has a relatively mild hearing loss is to try to cheer up the parents by saying it could be much worse. First, it is always a mistake to try to cheer up people in pain because it invalidates their feelings. The message received is that they have no right to feel badly. Second, the degree of disability is always in the eyes of the beholder. To these parents, the disorder is very severe, and their feeling needs to be respected and not minimized. At this point, the parents need someone to listen to them nonjudgmentally, someone who is not trying to focus their attention on content that they cannot absorb.

I leave parents of newly diagnosed children with the name and phone number of parents of an older child with a hearing impairment (they seldom call at first, as they are still in denial), and I set up an appointment to see them within a week. I may reframe the situation for parents by saying that they are now guaranteed to have an interesting life—not the one they thought they were going to have, but an interesting one nonetheless. In subsequent appointments I supply more information as the parents ask for it and seem ready to receive it. I start each session with that same question, "What do you need to know now?" I have found that the parents eventually ask all of the important questions. They might not be in the same order that would occur if I were in complete control of the content, but the important issues are covered. Parents ask each question when they are ready for the answer. Although it may take a bit longer to get the hearing aid on the child or to have the child enrolled in an educational program than if I had taken initial control, he or she will get there nonetheless. What is important is that the child gets there with parents who have taken responsibility and have actively participated in the educational decisions and are, therefore, more likely to follow through on good educational management practices.

Speech pathologists can conduct diagnostic evaluations of children in the same way. For example, in a speech or language evaluation, parents can be enlisted as codiagnosticians and experts on their child's behavior, and they can score the test results or elicit responses from the child. This empowers as well as educates the parents. For adult patients, it is necessary to empower the spouse (or significant other) as well as the client. I always bring spouses into the audiometric test booth and sometimes have them give the hearing test or mark the audiogram. Clients always select their own hearing aids and guide all aspects of their testing. Rollins (1988) has been conducting examinations of aphasic patients with the spouse as the active tester and the speech pathologist as the "coach." The "counseling" becomes much easier when the family participates actively in obtaining the diagnostic information.

One question that emerges very quickly once the diagnosis is agreed upon is the cause of the disorder. Handling this question is a very delicate counseling issue. One must determine responsibility without affixing blame. Parents who are obsessed with finding the cause are usually obsessed with guilt. They are looking to find a "cause" that is not their guilty secret. Each parent may be looking to blame the spouse or anyone else. It is very tricky handling this situation, and the careful clinician must steer a course between the Scylla of blame and the Charybdis of uncertainty. In order to have a successful outcome, parents must give up the past and the search for the cause and deal constructively with their "now." It is often fruitful to begin to explore the guilt issue at this time, although it may be hard to elicit. I have found that a rather neutral statement such as, "It must be so easy to feel guilty when you have had responsibility for bearing the child for so long," to be helpful to the mother, who is pressing me to find a cause for her child's deafness. I also tell her that she may have to learn to live with uncertainty as she may never know for sure what caused the child's deafness.

We often meet parents who don't seem to react at all to the diagnosis. In families in which a great many negative things have happened, the deafness is just one more thing. We recently had a family in the nursery in which the husband/father had left, and the mother and three children were now homeless and penniless. The mother had minimal physical and emotional energy to deal with her daughter's deafness. When told of the hearing loss, she responded with resignation.

People display their feelings in different ways. Some families and some cultures feel that it is inappropriate to display feelings publicly. These families seem to not react to the diagnosis although they may be deeply pained. Clinicians must not project themselves onto parents and expect all families to respond in the way they would if they had just found out that their children were impaired. It is very easy to get judgmental about families; this must be avoided at all costs.

I see the diagnostic occasion as the first step on the long journey that many clients have before them. If we do our job well, we can make that a giant step and help the clients avoid many pitfalls that await them. We can also make it much easier for the professionals who are further down the clients' habilitation road.

To summarize, there are seven steps needed for a healthy, client-centered diagnostic process.

1. Allow the client and family to tell their story. An open-ended question such as, "What brought you here?" is usually very helpful.

2. Enlist the family as codiagnosticians. Empower them with a statement such as, "You are the expert on this child, and I'll be the expert on the testing."

3. Involve the family and client actively in the testing procedure. The client should have choices where possible, and the family can be active in eliciting or scoring responses.

4. Have the client and family participate fully in the final diagnosis. In an ideal situation, they will make the diagnosis.

5. Empower them by asking, "What do you need to know now?" Let them guide you as to how much information you should give.

6. Listen and respond to the affect. Give clients a chance to talk about how they feel in an unhurried, caring atmosphere. If there is a time limit, then tell the family this at the outset, for example, "I have 15 minutes before my next appointment; how can I be helpful to you?"

7. Set up another appointment. Do not try to cover everything in one appointment. If this is not possible, help them locate additional support in the form of peer counseling.

6

Techniques of Counseling

I approach writing this chapter with some trepidation. If students concentrate solely on their counseling technique, their effectiveness can be severely limited. Good counseling technique flows from personality; it is seamless. Technique should not be readily apparent to the person being counseled or to an observer. This is not to say that there is no technique or that there is no discipline to be learned by the student. As the counselor gains more experience and becomes more secure, technique is incorporated into personality; the skill then becomes unconscious. I find that I frequently have to invent a reason why I did something when a student observer questions me in postevaluation sessions. Counseling is something I just "do"; if I am conscious of technique, I become mechanical and the technique fails because it interferes with the authenticity of the relationship. If the clients know they are being counseled, the counselor is probably doing it poorly.

Counseling is not a mantle that the professional puts on when a client is present and then discards the rest of the time. It is an attitude, something that is lived. I do not see how one can be a caring, responsive person only within the context of a client–professional relationship, and not in other aspects of one's life.

Counseling, as I view it, is an integrated approach to all interpersonal relationships; one "counsels" everybody who approaches in a caring and responsive manner. The techniques employed by a counselor will flow from personality and personal congruence, as well as from a counseling philosophy that has been incorporated into the way in which the counselor approaches clients. Each counselor develops a personal paradigm—a framework of thought, a personal strategy for understanding and explaining certain aspects of reality, a filter built from an individual's life experiences, prejudices, and constructs. A paradigm is the central organizer of how each person views reality. Events are filtered through our personal paradigms and interpreted by us. In counseling, our paradigms are influenced very heavily by our philosophical notions of how people learn.

In Chapter 2, I discussed four somewhat different ways of viewing the client. The behaviorist sees the client as a mass of conditioned responses; the humanist sees an organism that is seeking to grow; the existentialist sees someone struggling with the great issues of existence (death, freedom, loneliness, and meaninglessness); and the cognitivist sees someone who has made unfounded intellectual assumptions about the world that need to be examined.

Technique should not be bound to a particular philosophy. Although I like to think of myself as a humanist, I use some techniques that fit well within behavioral or rational–emotive therapy. I think a professional should not make therapeutic choices because of identification with a particular therapy, but rather because the evidence based on clinical experience has tended to indicate that this is the way to be most helpful to the client. Arbuckle (1970) wrote the following passage about this subject:

> In the long run, it would seem that the effective counselor is one who has worked out for himself, through the experience of experimentation, the means by which he can most effectively use himself in the human interaction known as counseling. His orientation has been eclectic, rather than parochial and while his own life is in a constant state of movement and change, he has learned that there are certain modes of operation which are most effective for him, thus there is a degree of consistency in his operation as a counselor. While he is open to consider any means that will work with the client he is aware that his own limitations are such that he cannot be all things for all people. He is acceptant of the thought that there is no model, no method, no technique, which will be consistently successful for him with any other human individual who may come to him as a client. (p. 291)

Counselor Control Via Response

In a counseling relationship, I wait to hear what issues are on the client's mind before I make a clinical judgment of how best to proceed. There are no stupid questions, only ill-judged responses. The nondirective or person-centered approach affords a great deal of counselor control. The way the counselor elects to respond will to a large extent determine the future course of the counselor–client interaction. The timing of a response is critical: Sometimes a client can make good use of content, and other times the content is very inappropriate. The counselor needs to select which response would be most facilitative within the context of client interaction. It is only through careful listening that the counselor can select the most facilitative response. If we listen carefully, the client will tell us what is needed.

A father of a deaf child might say, "There are no adequate services for deaf children in this state." I might respond to this statement in one of the following ways:

- Telling him about the services that are available and offering him a directory of services (content response).

- Asking him how he came to have that opinion (counterquestion).

- Commenting, "That must frighten you when you think about the available services for your child" (affect response).

- Telling him he is correct, and then commenting on what a wonderful opportunity this presents for him to get involved in establishing suitable programs (reframing).

- Telling him about my experience trying to find services for my child (sharing self).

- Responding with a clinical "uh huh" (affirmation).

None of these responses is necessarily the best one. (I have chosen six possible responses, which seem to me to be the most clinically facilitative.) Each response is appropriate within the context of the relationship. Each response will move the relationship into a different dimension, and the appropriateness is determined by a clinical judgment of the therapeutic context. The timing of the response is critical, as are many nonverbal features—tone of voice, facial expression, and body language. Let us look at each response in a bit more detail.

Content Response

The content response—the one most commonly used by professionals—generally keeps the relationship at an expected and rather predictable level. In the initial stages of a relationship, the professional provides content to establish credibility; in the latter stages, content is necessary for the making of appropriate decisions. Generally, content-based relationships are short term. When the professional has a limited amount of time, content predominates and tends to keep waiting rooms clear. A professional has the responsibility to keep current regarding his information and to separate fact from opinion—not an easy task. Content has immense value when it is used appropriately.

Counterquestion

I have found that people seldom want advice. They usually seek confirmation of a position or a decision that they have already made. Instead of revealing that decision, they often ask a question in hopes that I will confirm their position. Giving advice rarely works: A wise man doesn't need it and a fool won't take it. I have a sign over my desk that says, "Give me a fish and I eat for a day. Teach me to fish and I eat for the rest of my life." Advice giving is fish giving. People don't learn from it. If it works they are back for more, and if it fails they curse the giver of the advice, but in either case they have not learned. Often the most protective and facilitative response one can give to a confirmation question is the counterquestion.

The counterquestion forces the person to reveal his or her position. If one treats a confirmation question as a content question, then one is very likely to put one's foot in one's mouth. For example, a Spanish-speaking mother of a deaf son asked me whether she would she have to speak English to him at home if she enrolled her child in our nursery. I resisted the temptation to tell her that it would be less confusing for her child if she did (she could figure that out for herself) and instead responded by asking her what she wanted to do. The woman responded that if we made her speak English at home, she would not enroll in the nursery. I told her our policy was to speak English in the nursery and that she could decide what she wanted to do at home. The mother accepted that and a month later, when she was ready, announced to the parent support group that she was going to speak English at home. (At the time of admission to the program, she was not ready to give up her child as both a deaf child and a non–Spanish-speaking child. Parents will always find the "right" answer if we give them time and space to do it.)

It was a relief to me to realize that I did not have to answer questions. (I think this was a holdover from my school days when I was rewarded by answering my teacher's questions and thus could prove how smart I was.) The counterquestion is a very valuable teaching strategy. It forces the learner back onto his own resources. The counterquestion response to the client's lament, "You don't answer my questions," is, "Why should I answer your questions?"

Confirmation questions also are used to forestall rejection. A question is a low-risk contribution to an interaction: The questioner does not have to reveal himself or herself; instead he or she is asking the other person to make a revelation. For example, when I am asked if I am busy tonight, I usually respond by asking if the questioner had something in mind for me to do. Embedded in almost all questions is a statement, and I need to be sensitive enough to respond to the statement or at least to elicit it.

For me, the best indicator of the trust level in a professional–client relationship is the number of question–answer interactions. In initial stages of a relationship, where trust is not high, there are usually a great many questions. As the relationship develops and grows, the client becomes more willing to offer statements and observations. The professional can facilitate this therapeutic movement by not always answering questions and supplying content. The counterquestion can be a powerful tool for moving the relationship beyond the initial stages.

Affect Response

On the surface, the affect response appears risky, but actually it is responding to what Rogers in a lecture called "the faint knocking." By listening very carefully and trying to see the world as the client sees it and reflecting the feelings back, the counselor can help to open up the relationship—sometimes very dramatically. The appropriate affect response greatly increases the intimacy level in a relationship. I have found that even an inaccurate response is not harmful; it generally forces people to clarify further their feelings, and in the process of clarification, we both can generally understand the feelings better.

The affect response is very potent in building a counseling relationship. Caring is conveyed by our willingness to listen and be responsive to what the person says and also to what the person cannot quite bring himself or herself to say. Rogers (1951) called this *empathetic listening,* which at first glance would appear to be a readily teachable technique. Unfortunately, empathetic listening is often abused and can come across as parroting and mechanical in the hands of someone who has learned the form but not the substance of the humanistic approach. In an article written for physicians, Sabbeth and Leventhal (1988) talked about the "trial balloons" that patients and families send up when they interact with their doctor, asserting that it is the physician's responsibility to respond to the feelings imbedded in those "balloons." I remember one family that I worked with, in which the husband had had a severe stroke, and the wife said almost as an aside, "I can't seem to leave the house anymore without going back to check whether I have locked the door and shut off the stove. Sometimes I go back two or three times." My response to her was: "It seems like you don't trust yourself." This led to a very fruitful discussion of her anxiety and feelings of inadequacy in her ability to cope with her husband's disabilities.

The affect response requires considerable follow-up; it is rarely a response that one gives when there is limited time. I find that responding at the affect level is usually more appropriate in the initial stages of contact and diagnosis. It allows for a ventilation of emotions and for the alleviation of some of the secondary feelings that accompany the strong affect surrounding a catastrophic illness. The wife, for example, who feels very angry at her husband for having a stroke, can be given the opportunity to talk about her feelings of anger without feeling guilty. In later stages, when affect is not predominant, I generally give more content responses or reframe experiences into something more positive.

Reframing

The timing of reframing has to be precise and it cannot be used too frequently, or the professional will be accused of being a Pollyanna. It is immensely effective in mobilizing the person to look at the positive side. Good reframing always gives the person a jolt. It should cause the person to stop short and examine the assumptions underlying his or her statement. We as professionals are so focused on the problem that we seldom see the challenge that is present in the situation. Reframing encourages responsibility assumption. The parent who complains about the "dumb questions" he or she gets from strangers who see his child's hearing aids can be brought up short by the response, "What a marvelous opportunity to educate someone about deafness."

Professionals can also benefit from the reframing response by looking for the positive when analyzing their client relationships. For example, behavior can be interpreted as stubborn or as determined. If the clinician is always looking at the client's stubborn side, he or she will have a negative view of the client. A determined client has a much greater chance of success than a stubborn one.

I think that we seldom consider or call attention to a client's strengths, so often are we looking at the deficits. It helps, when I supervise student clinicians, to ask them, "What does this child have going for him?" and then, "How can we capitalize on those strengths?" When we focus on the client's strengths, somehow the problem begins to disappear far faster than when we emphasize the deficits. It might seem that there are limits to situations that can be reframed but that might not be so. I remember watching a video of Kubler-Ross counseling a woman in the terminal stages of amyotrophic lateral sclerosis (ALS). She was totally paralyzed and being cared for by her two daughters. Through one of her daughters, who bent close to her barely moving lips, she asked Kubler-Ross, "What good am I?" and Kubler-Ross's response, without batting an eye, was, "You are giving your daughters a chance to pay you back for all the care you gave them," which seemed to satisfy the woman.

I have several favorite reframings to the question, "Why me?" I might respond, "Why not you?" To families with children newly diagnosed as disabled, I might say, "This child has guaranteed you an interesting life." I try to reframe all "mistakes" into "nuggets of gold" whereby the person learned something valuable. I might comment to a client that his disability is a powerful teacher for him (and can be for others as well). I have personally found this notion of "teacher" in disability very potent. This notion also works with interpersonal and clinical relationships. I can reframe difficult clients into potent teachers for me, and I can do the same with previously obnoxious colleagues and acquaintances. If I approach them as people who have something to give me so that I grow, then the quality of the interaction changes markedly. For the astute businessperson, the complaining customer is his or her best friend, because that customer is helping improve the product. With such an attitude, you can change the world.

Reframing as a technique and as a life tool is very powerful. For all of the possible responses, but especially reframing, the timing is critical. It is very easy to lose people by reframing too early in the grief process; an ill-timed or ill-delivered reframing response can be very offensive. On the other hand, the ultimate goal of counseling is to help the clients reframe their life situations into something positive. When this is done by the clients themselves, the counselor's job is finished because there is no longer any problem.

Sharing Self

The image of the "professional" that most of us have is often of someone who is in total control at all times. This is someone who knows the answers and, therefore, is someone the client looks up to. In practice, we know that this is not true, that there are times when we (the "professionals") are out of control in our personal and professional lives. Standard clinical practice says we should hide this from our clients. I have found, however, that it is sometimes very helpful and facilitative to share our own doubts and uncertainties with clients. If we always seem in control, clients tend to feel very inadequate. A father of a child with Down's syndrome said, "I like to see the teacher have a hard time with my son. It validates my experience, too." Sometimes the most helpful thing we can say to a parent might be, "I haven't the foggiest idea what to do right now with your child. Do you have any ideas?" This empowers the parent and humanizes us at the same time.

Sharing self also means sharing our feelings by being willing to tell clients that we are angry at them. This is an opportunity to work out issues in the relationship. Few professionals ever let themselves be angry with clients directly. More often they ventilate on colleagues or repress the anger, which usually subverts the therapy. Similarly, we don't always share our positive feelings with clients. Sharing self reveals our authenticity as fellow human beings.

It is valuable to the clients to realize that the professional is also a person who has concerns, fears, and a life outside of the clinic. This revelation helps the client assume responsibility and prevents the professional from being elevated to the guru category. The timing of this response is especially critical. If it is done too early, the professional will lose credibility at a time when credibility establishment is critical for the relationship. The sharing responses should usually emerge later in the relationship and with clients who have a relatively high degree of self-esteem.

Affirmation

I am reminded of the countless cartoons featuring a psychoanalyst: A patient is on the couch talking and the psychiatrist is asleep; presumably progress is being made. Very often the client just needs a sounding board; he or she needs permission to talk and to express feelings without judgment. The "uh huh" response with appropriate nonverbal behavior can be very helpful in unleashing the client's feelings. The "uh huh" is also an affirmation that the counselor has heard the client, and an invitation for the client to continue. I have a poster in my office given to me by a group of students that says, "It often shows a fine command of language to say nothing." Sometimes the most facilitative remarks are the ones that you do not deliver.

The clinician has a wide array of potential responses; which one is selected can determine the direction of the client relationship. There are no "right" responses, only different roads to travel. If the response you give moves the relationship in a fruitful direction, then it is appropriate. It is also quite possible to recover from taking a less fruitful route. I have found that if something is important, it keeps coming up, and a feeling is seldom lost; it gets reworked and emerges again. The reader is reminded again that the nonverbal elements in interactions also are important, perhaps more important than what is actually said.

The following selected questions and statements were made by clients and/or family members. The reader may want to use them to practice the various responses discussed in this chapter. Again, there are no right or wrong answers, but different responses will accomplish different results.

1. If this were your child, what would you do?

2. Are cochlea implants any good?

3. My husband's family is very unemotional.

4. Will I have to be present when you test my husband?

5. Is it true that graduates of schools for the deaf are only able to read on a third-grade level?

6. What causes stuttering in a child?

7. Is the school for developmentally delayed children a good school?

8. Do we have to drill on the [s] sound any more?

9. My wife can't stand the sound of the artificial larynx.

10. I am so afraid of making a bad decision for this child.

11. You don't answer any of my questions.

12. I often think about my husband dying.

Hypothetical Families

The hypothetical families presented here are fictionalized case studies designed to illuminate particular problems. I have used them in classes I teach to speech pathology majors, in inservice workshops, and less frequently in parent groups. I found them very useful for me in my early work with groups when I needed the comfort of more structure and direction in my role as the leader. I seldom use them now because I prefer a much less structured experience.

The first 10 of the following case studies have been reprinted from a *Volta Review* article (Luterman, 1969). The case studies can be rewritten (I have done this with several) to reflect any disability. The original cases all involved deafness, but the problems illuminated by the case studies are universal. Interested readers may use the cases as is or may alter them to suit the needs of a particular group.

1. Mrs. A. is very confused. She has taken her two and a half-year-old son, who is neither talking nor seeming to respond to sound, to several physicians. Her pediatrician has told her that he thought her child was deaf but that nothing could be done until he was four years old. One physician has told her that he thinks the child is mentally retarded. Her husband and her in-laws, on the other hand, feel that there is nothing wrong with the child, and that he will "outgrow it." They tell her about an uncle who did not begin talking until he was four years of age and who is now perfectly normal. What should Mrs. A. do?

2. Mrs. B. sometimes says to herself, "Why did this happen to me?" She has said, "I know I shouldn't feel this way, but I really resent having a deaf child. He takes so much of my energy and time. He is so difficult for me to control; I worry about him so much. Every now and then, I find myself wishing for a moment that I had never had him, and then I feel guilty about feeling that way. I also hate to go out with him because of his screaming and because of the stares of passersby when they see his hearing

aid. I just can't stand the questions of strangers and their well-meaning advice any longer." What can be done about Mrs. B.'s feelings?

3. Mrs. C. feels that her deaf child was given to her because of her past "sins." She has devoted herself to taking care of her child; she no longer goes out socially and has dropped most of her friends. She spends a good part of the day working with the deaf child and taking him to his therapy lessons; she spends evenings reading and talking about deafness. She does not trust any babysitters. Mr. C. has begun to complain about feeling neglected and he says he is concerned about the two older children, who have not received much attention from their mother. What are your feelings about the C. family?

4. Dr. D. is a physician whose father and grandfather were also doctors. He has always wanted to have a son who would be a physician, too. Since he has learned that his only child is deaf and therefore will never be able to be a physician, Dr. D. has not devoted much attention to the boy. He has said, "I had so many plans for him. Every time I see the hearing aid it reminds me that he won't be what I would like him to be, and it's really very hard for me to be with him. I know I shouldn't feel that way and it probably is harmful to him, but having a deaf son is a very big disappointment to me." What can that father do?

5. Mr. and Mrs. E. have three children. Their youngest is a two-year-old deaf child; the other two are six and ten years of age. The E.'s have been very busy taking the two-year-old to various clinics for evaluations, and they have begun a twice-weekly therapy program and lessons at home. The middle child has responded to his younger brother's problem very well and, in fact, seems more understanding of it than the oldest boy. The oldest child has reacted with a great deal of jealousy. He is extremely difficult to manage; he throws violent tantrums and often simply withdraws for fairly long periods of time. Mr. E. has reacted to that behavior with stiff disciplinary measures. Mrs. E.'s reactions have varied from anger to pleading and bribing. At the same time, she recognizes that neither she nor her husband is handling the ten-year-old effectively. What might they do?

6. Mr. and Mrs. F. have a two-year-old deaf son. Mrs. F.'s parents live very near them, and Mrs. Z. has not accepted the fact that her grandson is deaf and will "never" be able to hear. She keeps sending her daughter articles from newspapers and magazines about operations and cures for deafness. She is constantly urging her daughter to take him to one more doctor. Mrs. F. says, "It is hard enough for us to accept our child's deafness, but it is especially difficult when we keep having to explain it over and over again to other people who don't really listen to us." Mr. F.'s parents, on the other hand, live farther away and see their grandchild rather infrequently. When they do see their grandson, they feel he should not be punished—"After all, he is deaf." They become upset if either Mr. or Mrs. F. disciplines the

deaf child in their presence. How could that family be helped to reduce some of these conflicts?

7. Timothy G. is a three-and a half-year-old deaf child with no siblings. He is not permitted outside the house unless accompanied by one of his parents, despite the fact that he lives on a quiet suburban street. His mother is very concerned that he might be hit by a child on a bicycle or by a car because he cannot hear. The parents are also afraid that he might fall down and hurt his ear with the hearing aid. Consequently, he seldom leaves his home or plays with children his own age. Should that situation be altered? Why? Why not? If so, what suggestions would you make to the parents?

8. Mr. and Mrs. H. live in a medium-sized town, 40 miles from Boston. They have lived in the town all their lives; Mr. H. owns and operates a small business there. The H.'s own their home in the community and they are both very active in community affairs. They have three children, aged ten, eight, and five, the youngest of whom is deaf and has been accepted in a school for the deaf in a suburb near Boston. Because of the distance involved, the school will accept the child only on a residential basis. Rather than have her daughter board at the school, Mrs. H. wants to move to a community close to the school so that her daughter can attend on a daily basis. Mr. H. is opposed to such a move; he feels that moving to the new community would disrupt the whole family. What should that family do?

9. Mr. and Mrs. I. find themselves at complete odds over the management of their deaf three-year-old son. Mrs. I. is convinced of the worth of the aural–oral approach and is trying to teach her son to lip-read and communicate orally. Mr. I., on the other hand, is convinced that only a very small percentage of deaf persons ever attain reasonable oral communication skills. He would prefer that his son learn manual communication, so he can at least communicate easily with other deaf persons. Mr. I. is around his children very seldom, but whenever he is, he uses manual signs to communicate with his deaf son. What can these parents do?

10. Mr. and Mrs. J. have a three-year-old deaf child. The family lives on an island and, because of the lack of facilities and professional help, Mrs. J. has had the sole responsibility for teaching her daughter. The child is doing well; she lip-reads about 30 words at this time, responds very well to contextual cues, and can use about 15 words expressively. Mrs. J. has placed her child in a nursery school with hearing children, where she also does well; she has just been told that her daughter can begin attending a school for the deaf on the mainland, which means that the child can get home only every four to six weeks. What should she do?

11. Mr. and Mrs. K. have recently divorced. Mrs. K. has retained custody of their three-year-old autistic son. The court has given Mr. K. permission to visit the child once a week. Mrs. K. finds that her ex-husband's visits are very unsettling to both her and their son. She feels that her son cannot

understand why his father leaves and is not home during the week; the child is very confused by the whole situation. Mr. K. also brings a great many presents when he comes, and takes the child to exciting places; by contrast, Mrs. K. feels that she looks very "bad" to the child and she is upset at the unfairness of the arrangement. What can this family do to relieve some of the tensions?

12. Mr. and Mrs. L. recently attended an IEP meeting at which the presiding educators unanimously voiced the opinion that their three-year-old child should go to the local school for the deaf. However, that school only offers a program in total communication. The child has been attending an aural–oral nursery school and has been doing quite well in developing his speech and language skills. The parents want him to continue in the aural mode and would like their child to attend a hearing nursery and receive tutorial help. They feel that the educators are suggesting the school for the deaf because it is expedient and not because it is the best facility for their child. The first IEP meeting ended in a deadlock, and all parties agreed to meet again in two weeks. What strategies should the parents employ for the next meeting?

13. Mr. and Mrs. M. have recently found out that their two-year-old child is deaf. They have one other, older child who hears normally. Mrs. M. has a deaf brother and a deaf uncle; consequently, she feels somehow responsible for the child's deafness. Mr. M. has not been helpful. He also blames Mrs. M. for causing the child's deafness and has left all the responsibility for the child's education to her. On one level, Mrs. M. deeply resents having that responsibility; on another level, she accepts it as her "punishment." What can Mrs. M. do to alter the unhealthy home situation?

14. The 11-year-old child with cerebral palsy of Mr. and Mrs. N. is deeply resentful of being disabled. He is constantly questioning Mr. N. about why he is disabled and refuses to believe that he will not outgrow it. He is currently being mainstreamed and is doing quite well academically; however, he has few friends among the classmates and he does not want to have anything to do with other people with disabilities. What can Mr. and Mrs. N. do to help their son?

15. Mr. and Mrs. O. are a couple in their 30s who have recently adopted an 18-month-old child, only to discover that the child is multiply handicapped. The adoption is not yet official, and the parents have the choice of returning the child to the agency and going on the waiting list for another child. Mrs. O. wants to keep the child because she has grown attached to him and feels that she can be a good parent of a child with disabilities. Mr. O. believes that they should return the child to the agency before they get any more attached. He feels that being a parent is hard enough and that being the parent of a child with disabilities is asking for too much trouble. He is not sure he has the resources to be a good parent to

that child, and Mrs. O. feels she cannot raise the child without the full support of her husband. What can that family do?

Locus of Control

Central to all counseling techniques is the notion of locus of control. Rotter (1966), a social psychologist, developed a scale that measures whether an individual has an internal or external locus of control. According to Rotter, people with an internal locus of control tend to feel that they have personal power and can control their own destiny. On the other hand, people with external locus of control feel that they are controlled by others. "Externals" believe that things just happen to them as the result of luck or fate. "Internals" feel their lives are "them doing them." Locus of control is conceived of as a continuum, with most people located between the extremes of total control (inner locus) and total powerlessness (external locus). Counseling technique, I believe, has to cede control to the client so that ultimately the client feels responsible and powerful.

Because behaviorists view clients as a mass of conditioned responses controlled by others, behavioral counseling techniques, if used too extensively and inappropriately, tend to encourage clients to have an external locus of control. A careful behavioral counselor teaches the client to identify the reinforcers in the environment and then teaches counterconditioning techniques. Clients in the hands of a competent behavioral therapist can develop an inner locus of control.

Within the sphere of humanistic counseling, control is always vested in the clients, making it easier for them to develop an inner locus of control because they have been given control over their learning from the inception of therapy.

The concept of locus of control has received some research attention in communication disorders. Dowaliby, Burke, and McKee (1983) modified the Rotter (1966) scale for use with deaf subjects and found that students with hearing impairment entering college were substantially more external in their locus of control than a control sample of students with normal hearing. White (1982) reported on a series of workshops he conducted with 281 teachers and counselors at six schools for the deaf. The participants were asked to rank 24 social competencies on the basis of what deaf children need to accomplish most. Almost all participants rated "accepting responsibilities for own actions" as the most important issue for deaf students. Bodner and Johns (1977) used the Rotter scale on 38 deaf students and found that they were significantly more external in their locus of control than the subjects with normal hearing.

The failure to take responsibility for one's actions in the adult deaf population was recently and vividly brought home to me. I lectured at a conference attended by a large number of deaf adults and my speech was interpreted. After the speech, which was an hour long, a deaf adult who was sitting in the back of the room complained vigorously that he missed the entire speech because he could not see the interpreter. The conference organizer, to whom I spoke afterward, felt guilty about the incident until we talked about it. She then realized that the responsibility was not hers. The deaf man could have moved his seat or complained at the onset of the lecture and the interpreter would have moved. Instead, he made a choice to sit there and then complain about it.

Locus of control has also been studied in stuttering populations. Craig, Franklin, and Andrews (1985) used the specially constructed Locus of Control of Behavior Scale on 17 stutterers in therapy. The researchers found that clients who moved toward internality in locus of control were more likely to maintain improvement over time. Relapse was more likely for those who did not internalize. Madison, Budd, and Itzkowitz (1986) found that stuttering children who showed greater internality also showed greater improvement following treatment than those children with a relatively external locus of control.

Locus of control has not been adequately researched in training programs. Only one study stands out. Shirlberg et al. (1977) examined locus of control in communication disorder majors. They found that students who have an internal locus of control were rated as the better clinicians. As they so aptly wrote, "Excellent clinicians do in fact view themselves as pilots rather than pawns of their fate" (p. 315).

Populations with disabilities have also been studied in regard to locus of control and, as one might expect, they have generally been found to have an external locus of control. Hallahan, Gasar, Cohen, and Tarver (1978) found that 28 matched teenagers with learning disabilities were significantly more external in their locus of control orientation than were control subjects. Land and Vineberg (1965) reported that blind subjects were more externally oriented then their sighted controls.

The finding of external locus in populations with disabilities is not surprising when one sees how professionals tend to interact with them. It is not uncommon to see professionals who are constantly "rescuing" clients: They are doing "Annie Sullivan." They don't want clients to experience additional failure or pain. In doing this, however, a clinician promotes an external locus of control that makes populations with disabilities— already dependent for so many things—feel that others are more powerful and more capable than they are.

Encouraging a more internal locus of control in our client populations is as much a matter of attitude as it is of clinical technique. The attitude we must convey to clients is that they are capable and that they have control of many aspects of their lives. The notion that the client always has control of how he or she will react to the disability is a paramount one. (Although a person may have no choice about being deaf, he or she always has a choice about what to do about the deafness.) The clinical techniques employed in helping clients should generally be covert and not obvious to clients or to observers. Many times we can be most helpful by not doing anything except being there as responsive, caring human beings, allowing the clients to work things out for themselves. Sometimes the very effective clinician creates vacuums that the clients have to fill, thus forcing clients to act and to take responsibility for their actions; in so doing, there is growth. Lesson plans, for example, need to be mutually arrived at with the client participating fully in planning the course of therapy. Asking children what toys they would like to play with or, as mentioned previously, when completing diagnostics, asking the clients what they need to know invests some control in them. In group meetings (discussed in the next chapter), I never call on participants; they are allowed to sit quietly as long as they like. The clinical silence or vacuum becomes a powerful teaching tool that, unfortunately, is not always appreciated by supervisors.

Language changing is a cognitive technique based on the rational–emotive therapy developed by Ellis (1977), which is more fully described in Chapter 2. Language changing derives from the clinical applications of general semantics. In this technique, the professional pays careful attention to the client's language, which illuminates the underlying and sometimes irrational assumptions the client is making. I have a poster in my office that says, "The shape of my world is the shape of my language." During an interaction I sometimes gently point out to the client the assumption underlying the words he or she is using. For example, the use of "have to" almost always reflects an external locus of control. When a parent said to me, "I have to try acupuncture," I said, "Don't you mean 'choose to'?" and a bit later, "Why do you feel you have to?" This was an invitation for the parent to look at the feeling of being driven and controlled by others. In this particular case, her own guilt was driving her. "But" always reflects an underlying ambivalence; I might respond to a statement such as, "I want to speak in public but I am afraid," with the response, "Can't you be afraid and still speak in public?" This encourages acting in the face of fear; the "but" allows wallowing in ambivalence. I always examine carefully all the "Yes, . . . but . . ." statements, which reflect ambivalence. "Should" and "ought" reflect guilt and deficiency. There is always some felt sense of failing when these words are used. Constructs such as, "I should talk to my pediatrician about his misdiagnosis of my child's hearing," might receive a response such as, "Do you want to talk to your physician?" "Should" and "ought" are also very reflective of an external locus of control, and changing them to "choose to" or "choose not to" encourages a more internal locus and assumption of responsibility for behavior.

We need to help clients recognize the choices they are making. I always examine the clients' language to see where they are evading responsibility. Evasion happens frequently when clients use the pronoun "we" instead of "I," as in, "We are unhappy with this class." I might respond, "Do you mean you are unhappy?" One indicator of a shift in locus of control is the spontaneous use of the "I" form, which reflects ownership of behavior. When that occurs in clients I know that we are well on our way to a successful counseling interaction.

When someone says she has been "lucky," I might change the word to "good." If a client says, "I was lucky to have him for a husband," I might respond, "You were good, so therefore he married you." It is very helpful to take credit for the good we do; most "lucky" people take all the responsibility for the bad and very little credit for the good. This is a hard way to live.

I don't allow clients to use collective nouns, such as "men" and "women." When I hear a sentence such as, "All men are lousy," I change it to "The men in my life have been lousy," and then I might gently comment, "It sounds as if you have not been meeting the right men." (I also might comment, "You sound pretty angry.")

Linguistic changes need to be made gently. The timing is critical. I seldom make linguistic changes in initial stages of diagnosis or when affect is high because changing languages forces the client into a cognitive stance. The client's trust in the professional also needs to be high, or the linguistic alterations can be seen as interfering and annoying.

Silence

Silence is an important component of any therapeutic relationship. A long, embarrassed silence frequently occurs early in my clinical interactions. Because clients generally expect me, the professional, to direct conversation, when I do not take the lead, a silence ensues. It is vital that I do not break this silence. It tells the others that if they want something to happen in this relationship, they have to act. The silence is a primary vehicle for responsibility assumption, and it is vital that I do not take that responsibility from the clients. Discomfort with silence initially forces many young clinicians to act; they then become role bound to make things happen while the clients sit back and watch.

Silences are generally uncomfortable in conventional relationships. I can remember the long painful silences I had as an adolescent on a blind date while I thought frantically of something to say. (I suspect the girl was adults at an early age; and this is something that many of these children seem to accomplish very well.

Grandparents

At this point in time, there is very little published research about grandparents. They often play a very important role in the families that we encounter, but they appear to be a badly underresearched, underutilized resource to the family and to the professionals.

The grandparents are present in every family whether or not they are actively involved. We always carry our family of origin into our new nuclear family. Our notions of what constitutes marriage and parenthood stem from our childhood experiences when we observe and assess our parents' parenting and our parents' marriage. We carry that image with us when we start our new family, either by imitating our parents or by being determined to be different. In either case, we are heavily influenced by them. Only with time and thought do we begin to find our way into marital and parental roles based on our own direct experiences. Some of the change comes about in the initial phases of family formation due to the stress of melding the spouses' disparate personal paradigms into the new family paradigm. Our ideas of what is appropriate and normal stem from our experience in our families of origin and reflect the values of our grandparents.

Grandparenthood is the ultimate developmental phase of parenthood. It is being able to parent without having the responsibility. Probably the one place that the child can have unconditional love is with the grandparents. Parents, because of their civilizing–instructing function, are often in conflict with their children. Grandparents generally have a more loving and accepting relationship with the child. I always knew that if the police were on my tail, my grandmother would take me in. My parents would also take me in, but they would believe the police. My grandmother would always believe me. A cynic has commented that grandparents and grandchildren are natural allies because they both have the same enemy. It is a rare person who has a bad relationship with his or her grandparent.

Unfortunately, the grandparent seems to be rapidly disappearing as an involved member of the family. Kornhaber and Woodward (1985) reported on their interviews of 300 grandparents and grandchildren. They found that only 15% of the families included an actively involved grandparent. The majority (70%) of grandparents were intermittently involved and 15% were not involved at all. The authors of the study felt that a new social contract was in effect that allowed the parents to define the grandparents' role, and the new role diminished grandparent involvement. (I think that the increased affluence that has enabled grandparents to live independently and at a distance from their children also contributes to this diminishing involvement. Extended families used to be a necessity because grandparents could no longer support themselves after retiring; Social Security has changed this.)

Based on their in-depth interviews of the children and the grandparents, Kornhaber and Woodward (1985) found that families benefited from closely connected grandparents. The grandparents functioned as mentors, caretakers, and mediators between the child and the parents; as sex role models; and as family historians. The results of this study suggested no negative effects of grandparent involvement. A different picture might have emerged if the authors had interviewed the parents, because grandparents can and frequently do introduce stress in the home.

There is minimal information in the literature about the grandparent role in families with a child who is disabled; they are generally the forgotten people. For example, a recent monograph published by the *Volta Review* with the title of "Families and Their Hearing Impaired Children" (Atkins, 1987) has no chapter devoted to grandparents.

Harris, Handiman, and Palmer (1985) used a questionnaire to interview the parents and grandparents of 19 children with autism. They found that the grandparents had a consistently less pessimistic view of the child's limitations than did the parents. They also noted that grandparents tended to deny the child's disability long after it had been accepted by the parents. Lowe (1989) adapted the Harris, Handiman, and Palmer questionnaire for grandparents of 39 deaf children. She found similar results, with the grandparents consistently more optimistic and more locked in denial than the parents.

These are the only two empirical studies in the literature concerning grandparents of children with special needs. They both validate my own clinical observations that grandparents generally lag behind the parents in accepting the disability. It is very difficult for the grandparents to deal with the pain of having a grandchild with a disability in conjunction with the pain their own child is experiencing. For the grandparents it is a double hurt, at a time in life when they are least prepared to cope with emotional emergencies. The grandparents, like most nonprofessionals, lack information and knowledge about the child's disorder. Consequently, their own children frequently know far more than they do, and a role reversal suddenly occurs. The parents, through their professional contacts and by virtue of living with the problem on a daily basis, generally move through the mourning stages much faster than the grandparents can. When we are hurting, we generally want and need support from our own parents. The parents of the child with a disability, when they seek support from their own parents, often find it is not there. Instead, the grandparents are seeking information and support from their own children. The parents are then in a role reversal where they are forced to parent their own parents. They often feel cheated and deeply resentful of this reversal because they themselves want badly to be parented, and the support is not forthcoming.

The parents are also plagued by feelings of guilt vis à vis their own parents; one of the "tasks" of children is to produce grandchildren for their parents; it is part of an implicit and sometimes explicit compact that parents and children have. When the parents have a child with a disability, causing their parents pain instead of joy—the parents may feel guilty. Anger very often masks the guilt that the parents feel and there is usually a very unhealthy dynamic that begins to develop in the parent–grandparent relationship.

Grandparents' feelings parallel closely the parents' responses. They feel grief, anger, anxiety, and guilt in varying proportions. They display their feelings to their children and to professionals in accordance with the cultural values of their family. More often than not, there is no openness about feelings between grandparents and parents. Frequently, neither wants to burden the other with their pain; they are very protective of each other. Unfortunately, this can be misinterpreted as indifference. Grandparents can be mistakenly viewed as being cold and uninvolved, when in reality they are frightened and concerned but very diffident about sharing their feelings. The parents and grandparents often need help in bridging the gap between them.

In the Emerson College program, we always try to provide a support group for grandparents, usually the most isolated and loneliest family members. It is difficult to assemble enough grandparents to have a group, since many grandparents now live long distances from their children and grandchildren and visit only intermittently. Nevertheless, we make the attempt every year by scheduling a nursery day on a Saturday, long in advance and in the spring when grandparents are more likely to return to the north, in the hope that we can gather enough grandparents for a group. I really enjoy a grandparent group, not only because I can relate so well to them since we are at similar life-cycle points, but also because of how lonely they are and how much they need support from us and from each other.

Occasionally all the grandparents live in our local area. When this happens, we offer the group an evening meeting in which I use the fishbowl design. Groups such as these almost invariably spark a great deal of family dialogue. They are also the most professionally satisfying groups that I lead.

The effects of the child with a disability on the parent–grandparent relationship does not have to be negative. Occasionally we have found the grandparents to be more capable than the parents, and they have assumed the primary caretaker role. They respond like parents, the only difference being that they are somewhat older and wiser; they are generally quite delightful to work with.

Parents frequently discover, after they have worked through their pain and anger, that the child's grandparents are an important resource for them, although not in the way that they had originally expected. Grandparents frequently provide respite care via very necessary babysitting so that parents can have some time out. Grandparents can also provide very necessary parenting to the other siblings in the family when the parents are overwhelmed by the demands of the child with a disability. The surrogate parent role played by the grandparents can become very important for the emotional well-being of the nondisabled siblings. The restructured relationship between the parent and grandparent, once the parent gets through the existential crisis, can also be very exciting. For the first time, the parents can begin to feel and respond as adults with their own parents and, in turn, find themselves being treated as adults.

Siblings

Siblings are enormously important for the development of social skills. Within the sibling system, children learn how to resolve conflicts and how to be supportive of one another. They learn how to make friends and allies, how to save face while losing, and how to achieve recognition for their skills. The sibling system teaches children to negotiate, cooperate, and compete. The jockeying for position within the family system shapes and molds children into their adult models. When children come in contact with the world outside the family, they take with them the knowledge they learned from their siblings to form their peer relationships (Minuchin, 1974).

The sibling relationship is potentially the longest relationship in our lifetime. In some families this relationship is fostered and strong; in others it is very weak. Siblings also serve to validate our growing-up experiences. No two children are ever born into the same family but the closest thing to someone who shares our cultural heritage is a sibling.

There is little in the literature about the effects of a child with a disability on the sibling system. Probably the most definitive study was by Grossman (1972), who tested and interviewed 83 college students who had siblings with developmental delay. She found that 90% of the siblings were affected by their developmentally delayed siblings. The 10% of the subjects who were not affected were the oldest male children. The most affected were the oldest sisters, who were expected to participate in childrearing activities and to assume many parental functions. In most families, there are different role expectations for oldest sons and oldest daughters. All younger siblings were affected one way or another by the child with a mental disability. The effects on the siblings were both negative and positive; in fact, the group of subjects split evenly, with 45% feeling that overall it was a negative experience and 45% feeling that it was a positive one.

The following negative consequences were noted by Grossman:

1. Shame about the developmentally delayed child, and guilt about that shame.

2. Guilt about being in good health while the sibling is not.

3. A sense of being tainted or defective: concern that they themselves might be mentally disabled or might bear disabled children.

4. Guilt about having negative feelings toward the sibling who is mentally disabled.

5. A feeling of having been neglected by the parents.

6. A feeling of having lost their own childhood because of the too-early assumption of responsibilities.

7. A belief that the child who is mentally disabled had put stress on the parental relationship, which negatively affected the rest of the family.

The positives for the siblings were the following:

1. Greater understanding of people in general and people with disabilities in particular.

2. More compassion.

3. More appreciation of their own good health and intelligence.

4. More sensitivity to prejudice.

5. A sense that the experience had drawn the family together.

6. A sense of vocational purpose and direction. (Many siblings become teachers of children with special needs.)

As one might expect, Grossman (1972) found that the more open and comfortable the parents were in talking about and accepting the child's disability, the better able the nondisabled sibling was to deal with it. When the parents accepted the child with a disability, they tended to help the nondisabled child also come to a healthy acceptance. This finding has strong clinical implications for professionals working with children with disabilities because by working with the parents, as system theory would predict, they can also be working with the sibling system. The other finding that needs to be emphasized is that as tragic as having a disabled child may be, it can and does have a very positive effect on some families and the children within the families.

Seligman and Lobato (1983) and Lobato (1983) reviewed all of the studies done on the nondisabled siblings of children with special needs. They concluded that there is a differential effect and called for longitudinal and better controlled studies. I fully concur with this finding. There are few studies of siblings within the field of communication disorders. All the studies I have found are within the field of deafness; one wonders how siblings of children with speech and language disorders fare. My experience would lead me to believe that there is no disorder-specific response and that all siblings will respond in pretty much the same way depending on the cues they receive from their parents.

Schwirian (1976) interviewed 29 mothers of families in which there was a preschool child with a hearing impairment with older siblings and 28 mothers of families with only nondisabled children. She found that older nondisabled siblings of children with hearing impairment children had greater care responsibilities and fewer social activities than older siblings in the control group. Sisters had significantly higher childcare and overall responsibility scores than brothers, again indicating the different role expectations that parents have for sons and daughters. A major procedural weakness of the Schwirian study is that she did not interview or test the siblings. Her data are only as good as the mothers are as observers of their children's feelings and behavior. In some cases, this may not be very ·accurate.

Israelite (1986) tested 14 hearing female adolescents (mean age of 16 years, 3 months) who were the older sisters of children with hearing impairment children and a matched group of 14 adolescents who had nondisabled siblings. All the tests used were self-report questionnaires. She found that the two groups differed significantly on only two traits, self-concept identity and social self. The results suggested that the hearing siblings defined themselves not only as individuals in their own right but as sisters of children with hearing impairment.

Darius (1988) interviewed siblings of children with hearing impairment. Her data indicated that siblings from small families, especially those with only two children, are most at risk for social and emotional difficulty. Siblings who are of the same sex and who are within two years of age of the deaf sibling are also at risk. Her data supported the notion that how well the parents accepted and adapted to the deafness was the major variable in the siblings' acceptance.

For my book, *Deafness in the Family* (Luterman, 1987), I interviewed some of the original families that had gone through the Emerson College program. In one family, the oldest daughter had become a speech pathologist in Hawaii. I wrote and asked her to write me of her experiences growing up with a deaf brother. I think her letter, printed below, poignantly illustrates the problems of the hearing sibling.

Dear Dr. Luterman:

I have been very busy this spring with work, my two special education classes that I am taking at the University of Hawaii, and the new group that I joined called Sign Express. It is a group of about 15 people that sign songs and put on performances to help educate others about sign language.

I am real excited about the book you are writing and I wish that I could have been there to talk with you when you went over to my family's house. I have a lot of feelings about Robert's deafness and how it has affected me. I have only told my mother some of my feelings because she gets upset or angry when I say how I felt when I was little. I don't know if it's because she thinks that I am saying that she was not a good mother to me, or why she gets upset.

I think when I was little, I had very mixed feelings. I felt very jealous of Robert but I also felt very proud of him. I can remember feeling very neglected, because I always thought that he got all of the attention from everybody. Of course now I realize that my mother had to work with him more and it was all necessary, but I didn't understand that when I was little. I remember wishing that I was deaf for a while thinking that then I would get more attention. I remember wishing that I would get sick and have to go into the hospital so that everyone would bring me presents and give me more attention. I even remember trying to break my arm by jumping out of my treehouse (which never happened). I have never told my mother any of this. But I never hated Robert. I guess the way I dealt with my jealousy was by deciding to work with deaf children when I grew up. I decided this ever since I used to go watch Robert at Emerson College through the one-way mirror with my mother. And here I am, a speech pathologist working at a school where the deaf total communication class is housed, and I love working with the deaf kids (ages 5–12).

I also remember being very proud of Robert. I can remember going to his school plays at the school for the deaf and having tears come to my eyes when I watched him on stage. I remember wanting to be friends with his friends there. I also remember people saying mean things about deaf people in general, like they can't talk and they are all "deaf and dumb," and feeling so hurt and intimidated that I couldn't even stand up for deaf people. I usually just said nothing.

I guess Robert's deafness probably created a lot of extra tension in my parents' marriage. I remember my mother getting really upset about the taxis taking him to school, some school problem, and other things. I remember my father not wanting or just not getting involved and my mother getting upset at him. I really never understood just how it affected my father but I know it was real hard on my mother. I never really noticed what effect Robert's deafness had on Lynda, Michael, or Nicole [siblings]. I didn't get along with Lynda, Michael, or Robert that much when I was little. Now I am much closer to everyone in my family.

Maybe it's because I live so far away. I am trying to learn to sign fluently. Robert prefers to sign now and doesn't associate with hearing people if he can help it. Last summer when I went home for a visit, I played the card game Uno with Robert and his friends. At first I felt uncomfortable, but it was a lot of fun and I think that was the first time anyone in our family associated with him when he had his friends over. I wish I could spend more time with him and really get to know him. I have been able to get a hold of a TTY a few times and I love being able to talk to him over the phone. I always felt bad when I called home on holidays and could talk to everyone and then just be able to tell someone to say hi to Robert. I remember a couple of times he would get on the phone to say hi to me and then my mother would get on the phone and say "that was Robert," like I couldn't tell. I remember when we used to watch TV when we were little and Robert would always ask us what was going on in the show and we would get irritated at him and tell him to wait for the commercials. I wish we knew how to sign then and be able to interpret for him so he could understand while the show was on. I have very strong feelings about total communication. Robert has told me a lot about how he always felt left out and that makes me feel so sad for him because if we only used sign language he would have been more involved and would have known what was going on. But I realize that is a big issue that probably never will be solved.

Well I guess I rambled on quite a bit. I hope that this information will be helpful to you. If you have any more questions, please feel free to write to me. I'll be glad to help in any way possible. I would love to visit you the next time I get back to Boston and also visit the clinic at Emerson College.

Thank you for asking [about] my feelings.

How often do we ask siblings how they feel or include them in what we do? They can be immensely helpful in conducting diagnostics and in administering therapy. I often use them as test models for their siblings with hearing impairment. In the nursery program, we always set aside several days each semester specifically for siblings. On these days, the hearing children are allowed into the nursery and the therapy sessions. We give them a hearing test so that they know what takes place in a test suite. We are always very careful to ask them if there is something they want to know. Very often the siblings are our future speech pathologists and audiologists.

At some point all parent groups in which I have participated have brought up the problem of siblings. It often occurs in the first meeting as parents are burdened with the guilty knowledge that they have been ignoring the hearing sibling in the family. The solution to the sibling problem is easy to grasp intellectually and very hard to implement practically.

Parents need to direct attention to the sibling as a person, not merely as a vehicle to produce a well-functioning child with a disability or as an impediment to that mission. Means must be found within the family for the sharing of feelings, and siblings must be given a chance to discuss their feelings of anger and guilt. Unfortunately, a fair balance is not easy to achieve, especially in the early years, as the parents do not have much energy and time for themselves, let alone for the nondisabled siblings. Parents frequently can identify the problem; however, because of limited resources, they cannot implement a solution. Here the grandparents can be very helpful. Also, paradoxically, if we can teach parents to take care of themselves, they will have the energy and time left to share with the nondisabled siblings. Parents don't always see that it is not the quantity of time they spend as much as it is the quality.

Optimal Families

When we broaden our view from individual therapy to family therapy as proposed here, we in effect become a member of the family. As a member of the family, we teach by modeling effective behavior. For us to do this, we need to have a grasp of what it is we are working toward to help the family become more optimal. Several models of the optimal family have appeared in the family literature (Beavers & Voeller, 1983; Epstein, Bishop, & Baldwin, 1982; Olson, Russell, & Sprenkle, 1983). From these studies I have distilled five characteristics of the optimal family.

Communication among all family members is clear and direct.   Almost any family therapist who has written about families has examined the communication patterns in the family. Invariably, dysfunctional families have dysfunctional communication patterns. Using modeling, therapists encourage clear communication. Optimal families do not hold back or talk around an issue. Implicit expectations are always made explicit. Comments are always directed toward the person for whom they are intended. Talking is efficient and straightforward. Messages are congruent, containing both content and feelings. Empathy and humor characterize the communication among family members.

Roles and responsibilities are clearly delineated, overlapping, and flexible.   An optimal family must have clear intergenerational boundaries, as well as a delineated sibling subsystem. The parents must have clear authority with other roles, which are allocated on the basis of ability rather than on the basis of age or gender. Roles need to be overlapping as well, so that if one member of the family is not present, others can fill in. The children's responsibilities need to be altered as they grow, and responsibilities need to be renegotiated periodically. There must be a basis and structure for negotiation of role allocation. Optimal families allow for change in roles as needed to maintain a well-functioning unit.

The family members accept limits for the resolution of conflict.   Conflict in families is normal and healthy; growth and change occur out of conflict. Parent–child and sibling relationships are inherently conflictual. In dysfunctional families, conflict is repressed; the family might appear harmonious, but when conflict does emerge it becomes destructive. In optimal families, disputes are resolved in a way that is mutually satisfactory, and there is always a face-saving formula for any "loser." Conflict in an optimal family usually involves everyone winning. For example, the mother is about to cut a cake and the children are squabbling over who is going to get the bigger piece of cake. The mother lets one child cut the cake and lets the other child choose the first slice; the other child will cut the next cake and the first child will choose. Children need to see that solutions are fair and that individual needs are always considered. Parents must also model conflict resolution for their children as the professionals model it for the parents.

Intimacy is prevalent and is a function of frequent, equal-powered transactions.   One basic function of the family is to provide an environment where members feel loved. Families have different ways of expressing love. Some express this love physically through hugging and kissing, whereas others use more subtle expressions of caring. The caring needs to be communicated in a way that the other family members can receive it. An optimal family provides intimacy while also respecting the need for space and distance. Optimal families are cohesive without being enmeshed.

A healthy balance exists between change and the maintenance of stability.   The maintenance of stability is known as homeostasis. Families maintain their balance by making minute adjustments much as a highwire performer oscillates movements to stay on the wire (Harvey, 1989). Families must change to accommodate the life cycle. For example, the children age and make new demands on the parental restrictions; meanwhile the parents age and are less adept at managing their lives, so other family members must fill the void. Then there are the vicissitudes of life when a family is thrown a "curve ball." This happens when parents get ill, when an economic catastrophe occurs such as the loss of a job, or when a child is born with a disability. Optimal families are able to make the necessary changes while maintaining stability. Dysfunctional families are not able to accommodate to the change, and often dissolve or become so dysfunctional that they need massive amounts of external support.

The delicate balance between homeostasis and accommodating to change involves all of the other factors involved in an optimal family. Change can be accomplished best where there is open and clear communication among the family members, and where role flexibility enables others to step in to accommodate the increased demands of family time. There needs to be caring among the family members, and the family needs to have a means of dealing with the conflict that is inevitable any time there is a need for change.

Optimal families produce optimally functioning children and adults with disabilities. Our job as professionals in working with persons with communicative disorders is to help the family become optimal, or as close to it as possible. We can teach parents, mainly by modeling, how to manage conflict, how to communicate openly and honestly with their children, and how to display their affection and caring for their children. In effect, what we must do is parent the parents and create for them in our relationship an optimal family. The parents then can take from our optimal clinical family the information and skills necessary for their own home situation.

The Successful Family

The notion of the optimal family is basically theoretical, stemming from the experience of family therapists working with dysfunctional families. There is some research on the successful family. The design of these studies was basically the same: The professionals working with the families rated the families as to their degree of success in coping with a child with a disability. Based on the ratings, the investigators then categorized families as successful, adequate, or inadequate. These families were then interviewed to determine the outstanding characteristics that led to the professional judgment. Gallagher et al. (1981) examined families in which there was a child with developmental delay; Lavell and Keogh (1980) examined families in which there was a child with diabetes; and Venters (1981) studied families in which there was a child with cystic fibrosis. The results of these studies suggest that four characteristics seem to underlie a successful family. These characteristics are very much in agreement with my own observations of the families of deaf children.

A successful family is one that feels empowered. Families need to feel that what they are doing will make a difference. Even with children having cystic fibrosis, a terminal illness, the parents need to feel that by working with the children they can prolong their lives and make their current living easier. I frequently see professionals who present such a bleak and hopeless picture to these parents that the parents never get over the feeling of

"What's the use." These families are never successful; we must never take away hope.

Parents are often rendered impotent by too much help from professionals. Sandow and Clarke (1977) studied the effects of a home intervention program on the performance of preschool children severly affected with Down's syndrome and severe cerebral palsy. The 32 children in the study were divided into two matched groups. One group was visited by a therapist once every two weeks for a two-hour session, whereas the other group was visited only once every two months. The study was conducted for three years, and at the end of each year the children were tested for their cognitive functioning and speech and language development. The findings were startling. Initially the more frequently visited children showed more gains in intellectual functioning and growth in speech and language than the less frequently visited children. By the second year of the study, the results reversed, with the less frequently visited children demonstrating more improvement than the more frequently visited children. By the third year, the gap had increased even further, demonstrating that less professional intervention was better than more. The researchers interpreted their data to suggest that parents in the less frequently visited group were less dependent on the therapist than were the more frequently visited parents. In short, they were empowered in that they were forced to rely on their own skills and strengths because they had a minimum of professional help.

My bias about home intervention programs is that they should be almost entirely parent centered and that the teachers should interact minimally with the child. The parent should do the lesson, and the teacher should focus on those things that the parent is doing well. The help provided by the teacher to the parent needs to be covert and not very apparent if the parent is to be empowered.

In successful families the self-esteem, especially of the mother, is high.   This notion is very much related to the empowering notion discussed above. I think that the single most potent clinical intervention we can make to help a young client with a disability is to bolster the self-esteem of the parents, especially the mother. There is research justification for this notion. In a hallmark study, Schlessinger (1994) followed 40 families with a deaf child on a longitudinal basis for 20 years. She found that the best predictor of third-grade literacy was the self-esteem of the parents. This variable transcended hearing loss, methodology, and socioeconomic status. This means that every clinical intervention that we perform needs to be evaluated in terms of whether or not it enhances the self-esteem of the parents. Efficacy of our clinical interventions is going to be a matter of parental self-esteem.

When parents feel confident and empowered, they no longer need denial as a coping strategy. They then are able to work with the professional as coequals. When this happens, the child benefits immensely. In the same vein, when working with adult clients, professional attention needs to be directed at empowering and increasing the self-confidence of the nondisabled spouse.

Therapists need to set up situations whereby the parents can experience some success in working with their children, especially in the early stages of the parent–professional interaction. As Featherstone (1980) so eloquently wrote, "Fears ease as experience discredits fantasy, as mothers and fathers learn that actual problems of raising their child differ from the ones they imagined. Similarly, small victories over private demons reassure parents about their own ability to raise their child" (p. 27).

In successful families there is a feeling that the burden is shared.   In most families one person, usually the mother or the nondisabled spouse, is designated as the primary caretaker/therapist for the person with a disability. If the rest of the family provides no support and respite care, the designated caregiver begins to feel resentful and martyred. When this happens, there is very little likelihood of a successful outcome. Other family members need not be overt in their help, but they need to be emotionally supportive of the caretaker and also be willing to assume some of the other family responsibilities, freeing the caretaker to provide the direct therapy. This can occur even in a single-parent home if there is a feeling of a supportive network around the primary caretaker. Friends and other family members can fill in for the missing parent. Dundon, Carmer, and Novak (1987) found that two major variables determining success of families coping with Alzheimer's disease was health of the well spouse and the amount of unpaid help available to the family; when the well spouse felt supported by the community, the family coped successfully.

The family also needs to feel that the larger community is supportive and is sharing the burden. In the initial diagnostic stages with a young child, the parents feel totally responsible. I often tell them, "This business is really in thirds—one third is your responsibility, one third is mine as a professional, and one third is the child's. You just be sure that you do your third, I'll do my third, and both of us will see that the child does his third."

Successful families need to make philosophical sense of the situation.
All of us have a cosmology that is our way of explaining why and how things happen, especially why bad things happen. It is hard for most of us to accept the existential notion of randomness or the concept that we live in a world without meaning. So people seek an answer to the question,

"Why me?" To not have a suitable answer may leave us stuck in bitterness and anger, which seldom leads to a successful outcome. Each family must come up with its own answer, which means that we as professionals sometimes need to get into uncomfortable areas of discussion as people come to grips with their own explanation of why the terrible thing happened to them. For example, in one support group, a parent of a deaf child said, "Since this happened, I have stopped going to church," and a mother sitting opposite her said, "Since this happened, I've been going to church every day." A very fruitful discussion then ensued, as the parents worked through their feelings toward "God" and reworked their religious views.

A very successful mother of two deaf children and one child who is severely brain damaged as a result of a car accident had this to say:

> I always think of myself as a very average person. I have no particular talent, no particular anything. I'm a very average type person and I've been given three very special kids. Sometimes I talk to God and I say, "Why did you give these kids to me? Why didn't you give them to someone who was different?" and so then I think, all right, I was given these kids and maybe this is my thing in life. Maybe all I'm going to do in life is to get these kids into adulthood, and maybe this is how my salvation will be measured.

With an explanation we can go on and work; without one we are forever pondering the why. For me, having a wife with multiple sclerosis is a challenge to make something good happen out of an awful disease. There is a marvelous Zen saying, "When the learner is ready, the teacher appears." For me and my wife, multiple sclerosis is our teacher.

The stress on families, which is both a reflection of sociological changes and the change engendered by a person with a disability, is not necessarily a negative force. I have seen a great deal of growth occur as a result of this stress. Many siblings decide to become therapists. Although some marriages founder, others are strengthened. For the parents, the child with a disability can offer an opportunity to restructure a relationship that has gone stale. Men have often reported how delighted they were to find out how much strength their wives have; the wives were delighted with the caring qualities that emerged in their husbands. Often both parents have found a new purpose in working very hard together in parent organizations and therapy programs, thereby strengthening the bond between them.

Similarly, the parent–grandparent relationship can be restructured. For the first time, many parents begin to respond as adults to their own parents and, in time, find themselves being treated as adults. They often begin to see their own parents as vulnerable fellow adults, and that is very exciting.

For me there has always been growth in stress. I am pushed by the stress to develop more capacity in order to reduce the stress. We generally give to life what life demands. When life demands more, I am forced to expand. That increased capacity is my growth. I see this happening in all the families I have worked with, and although I can empathize and perhaps sympathize with the pain involved, I know that if they can just hang in, they will learn and grow. They have a powerful teacher in the disorder; and we as professionals must allow the process of growth to take place. We can facilitate the growth by not overhelping; by at all times respecting the dignity and the capacity of our clients to grow. Very often we have to let go of our preconceived notions. The following anonymously written poem has helped me with the necessary letting go:

To Let Go

To Let Go is not to stop caring,
It's recognizing I can't do it for someone else.
To Let Go is not to cut myself off,
It's realizing I can't control another.

To Let Go is not to enable,
But to allow learning from natural consequences.
To Let Go is not to fight Powerlessness,
But to accept the outcome is not in my hands.

To Let Go is not to try to change or blame others,
It's to make the most of myself.
To Let Go is not to care for, it's to care about.
To Let Go is not to fix, it's to be supportive.

To Let Go is not to judge,
It's to allow another to be a human being.
To Let Go is not to try to arrange outcomes,
But to allow others to affect their own destinies.

To Let Go is not to be protective,
It's to permit another to face their own reality.
To Let Go is not to regulate anyone,
But to strive to become what I dream I can be.

To Let Go is not to fear less, it's to love more.

9

Counseling and the Field of Communication Disorders

Educating the Clinician

During the 1960s, a notable attempt was made to define the field of speech pathology and audiology by giving it a narrow, technical base. This insured our survival as an independent profession with a solid core of research expertise and scientific credibility. Now that we are established, we have been moving into a more humanistic, family-oriented field that borrows heavily from psychology, social work, and family therapy.

It presently appears that our training programs are lagging behind the needs of the field. As stated in Chapter 1, McCarthy et al. (1986) surveyed the ASHA-accredited training programs. They found that only 40% of training programs offered a course in counseling within their department, 36% offered a course outside the department (over half of these courses were offered within psychology and education departments and had no content related to speech and hearing), and 23% offered no course in counseling. Only one third of the programs require that students take a counseling course, despite the fact that 70% of the respondents felt that counseling was a very important skill that should be offered within the program. The authors concluded their study with the following observation:

> Although the fields of audiology and speech–language pathology recognize counseling as an essential component of diagnostic and therapeutic

procedures and as a professional responsibility, the emphasis training programs place on it may not reflect its importance. Students are often trained in counseling theory and techniques only when they have chosen to take such a course. Even then, counseling specific to communication disorders is frequently not included. These data are underscored by the finding that only 12% of the respondents in this study felt that training programs are sufficiently preparing students to meet the counseling needs of individuals with communicative disorders. (p. 52)

The follow-up to that study has indicated no essential change in our field (Culpepper et al., 1994). I, too, feel that we are not training our students appropriately to prepare them to meet the emotional demands of a helping profession. From the humanistic point of view, a client's learning and growth take place best in a nonthreatening atmosphere of warmth and acceptance. In order to facilitate this growth, the therapist needs to be a caring, nonjudgmental, congruent person. None of these skills is exotic; they are all within the purview of everyone. The job of the training program is to help develop these attributes in student clinicians. Unfortunately, almost all graduate training programs tend to stress the intellectual and cognitive skills of the students and do not emphasize their interpersonal abilities. For example, selection of students is generally based on the intellectual skills as exemplified by Graduate Record Examination scores or grade-point averages. Rarely are interpersonal skills considered, except perhaps indirectly as reflected in letters of recommendation. However, the present era of full disclosure and threat of litigation has rendered letters of recommendation almost meaningless. The grade-point average seems to lend an objective measure that we can defend. Interpersonal skills are not readily measurable and may be difficult to defend if challenged by an irate student. The danger for our field in ignoring interpersonal skills, however, is very great; we can turn out students who are knowledgeable about the field but who are clinically and interpersonally inept.

It appears that we are selecting reasonably "normal" graduate students. Crane and Cooper (1983) gave the Minnesota Multiphasic Personality Inventory (MMPI) to 130 female speech–language graduate students. They found that the resultant profiles "were manifestly normal but rather passive, compliant, stereotypically feminine, sensitive, anxious" (p. 139). It concerns me that we are willing to accept these attributes as normal for women. I prefer to think that much of what we are viewing as "stereotypically feminine" is in reality a reflection of our teaching and attitudes toward women. I hope that this attitude is changing. I am deeply concerned about the passivity and compliance aspects of the personality profile, and what that bodes for our profession. In all fairness, Crane and Cooper also found that our students were highly imaginative, creative, and energetic—and I have certainly met and worked with my share of students with these delightful characteristics. From the research of Miller and Potter (1982), however, we also know that many of these students will burn out at an alarming rate.

Training Students for Clinical Competence and Personal Growth

I am not sure that the MMPI measures some important personality variables that influence clinical competency. For example, the "Annie Sullivan" type of student needs to be identified early in his or her career. This type is a caring person with energy and a marvelous impulse to be helpful that can be directed, but we must provide experiences on the training level to increase self-awareness of the need to be needed. The Annie Sullivan types must learn how to help in a way that is truly helpful so that the client's self-esteem and independence are not compromised. Our personal satisfactions can come from knowing internally what we have done and not from receiving the approval of others. In short, we also have to help develop in students an inner locus of evaluation.

Occasionally we get interpersonally inept students who are otherwise quite bright, and there needs to be a place within our profession for them. I think they can be helped to become more adept with some structured interpersonal experiences; they may also make good researchers.

Another kind of student occasionally gets through our screening process: the student with a very limited capacity to care for others. I think that I can teach almost anything except the capacity to care. This student probably will be a professional disaster despite any technical skills we might teach, and we need to have better mechanisms to screen such students out of the profession.

If one examines closely the training of speech pathologists and audiologists, it is apparent that the training is along poorly conceived behavioral lines. Control is generally external to the students: The teacher decides what the students need to know and rewards them if they appear to learn the material. Student clinicians also learn to please the supervisor, which also encourages the development of an external locus of evaluation. (No wonder they are passive and compliant!) How often do students get a chance to select their own material to be learned, and how often are they required to evaluate themselves and perhaps their supervisor?

The communication disorders literature reveals a strong humanistic trend in the supervisory relationship. Ward and Webster (1965) urged that we treat our students as human beings, and that their self-actualization be an important consideration in the training program. They argued for courses within the curriculum that are geared to explain human behaviors and that can then be applied to students. Van Riper (1965) described the sometimes painful role of the supervisor:

> He is a friendly person looking on interestedly in what is taking place, warmly empathizing with the success and making no issue about the failures. Even when the student is demonstrating outrageous sins of omission or commission the supervisor does not seize the reins. He suffers silently and keeps a poker face and formulates what he will say to the clinician later. (p. 77)

Van Riper believed that we should treat the student clinician with the same loving respect that we wish him to accord the client.

Pickering (1977) argued that the student needs to have skills in relationship as much as knowledge about the field. She stated that the supervisory relationship can be the vehicle for the student to learn about relationships and for promoting personal growth and change in both the supervisor and student clinician. The supervisory relationship needs to have the elements of authenticity, dialogue, risk taking, and conflict in order to facilitate growth.

Caracciolo et al. (1978) wrote that a supervisor should model the Rogerian, nondirective role to the students. The Rogerian relationship would have a high degree of unconditional regard, empathy, and congruence. The students, after experiencing the growth in this humanistic relationship with the supervisor, would in turn be able to foster this kind of relationship with their clients.

I agree with the premise of Caracciolo et al. (1978) that experiencing the humanistic relationship is the best way of learning it. The authors make me uncomfortable, however, when they state that "it is necessary to define operationally and construct specific training procedures that will develop among supervisors the necessary attitudes and skills that will contribute to personal and professional growth" (p. 290). It seems to me that when we set about "operationally defining" and "developing specific training procedures," we lose the essence of the humanistic approach. At some fundamental level, humanism is ineffable. True learning is an inside-out process; we must lead students to it and hope they find it by creating for them the right conditions of a growth-promoting relationship. When we deliberately structure the learning situation so as to teach techniques, we are imposing a cognitive solution on an affect problem. Students tend to learn the form of the humanistic approach but not the substance. (Anyone who has tried to have a conversation with a student who thinks that Rogerian reflective listening means repeating back the last thing the person has said begins to get an insight into the causes of homicide.)

Klevans, Volz, and Friedman (1981) attempted to train students in interpersonal skills. One experimental group was taught skills via extended role playing, having to assume the role of a person with a speech, language, or hearing impairment in an out-of-class assignment. The second group was required to observe clinical interactions and to code behavior. The authors found that the students in the experiential group were able to make significantly more facilitative verbal responses than the coding–observing group when tested in a simulated helping relationship. The authors felt that the total length of time (8¾ hours) devoted to training both groups was insufficient for mastering interpersonal skills.

I think this study points up several things that need to be examined. If we are going to train students in interpersonal skills, the experience needs to be hands-on rather than didactic. We cannot lecture within a class or even have students observe interactions and then expect them to be interpersonally adept. It is also clear that we have to allot more time within the curriculum for working on interpersonal skills. The 8¾-hours of time allotted in this study, which was part of a one-credit clinic practice course, is unfortunately typical of most training programs and rather pathetic for attempting to teach such fundamental clinical skills.

I think we also need to attack the problem from the personal growth side. We cannot limit our endeavors to teaching interpersonal skills from a strictly technical point of view. For me, the best way of teaching and learning counseling has been within the context of my own personal growth experiences, which have included such diverse activities as attendance at workshops, immersion in sensitivity groups, and an Outward Bound learning experience where I had to rock climb and sail. The latter experience was especially helpful; an underlying theme of that experience was, "We have met the enemy and found it is us." I have found that as I have come to accept myself more, I also accept and value others more. I have had to learn to give myself permission to think, to feel, and to be productive.

The dilemma of the supervisory/teaching relationship in developing humanistic relationships with students is the evaluative function held by the teacher. As long as the supervisor/teacher has the power of the grade, locus of control is always external to the student, and authenticity on the student's part in relation to the supervisor is very hard to accomplish. At some level and at some time, the student must please the teacher in order to get a passing grade. It would require a very high degree of trust to develop authenticity in the relationship. True equality is not really possible because the levels of personal power are inherently unequal. Van Riper (1965) argued that we should be collaborators with our students rather than supervisors. This ideal is very hard to accomplish when the supervisors must give the students grades or eventually write letters of recommendation. Although the supervisors may feel that they are collaborators, the students feel differently. Culatta, Colucci, and Wiggins (1975) found wide discrepancies between the supervisor's and the student clinician's views of their relationship.

In my teaching of content-level courses, I have attempted to work out a compromise between cognitive and interpersonal learning needs. At the beginning of the course, I give the students the final examination, which consists of a list of essay questions that reflect my opinion as to what content they need to master and from which I will select some unspecified number of questions. I also give the students a bibliography containing readings that will enable them to find the answers to the questions. It is then the students' responsibility to organize their time to master that content. The grade for the course is based solely on the examination performance, and students are encouraged to be as ignorant as possible during class sessions. I comment that they should be ignorant; that's why they are taking the course. The only time they cannot afford to be "ignorant" is on the final examination.

I usually take responsibility for structuring half of the class sessions with lectures, films, videos, or guest speakers. The students are required to structure the other half of the sessions. The unstructured sessions usually start out with painful silences until the students realize that nothing happens until they make it happen. Periodically we evaluate the class, and everyone, including myself, has a chance to talk about how things are going. Within this format, the students get a chance to obtain some control of what they learn; they have to take responsibility for obtaining content and are never required to read anything. Generally the course evaluations by the students are enthusiastic, although as we near examination time, their anxiety begins to increase and they begin to have regrets about their freedom. Because the students are not usually familiar with a learning situation in which they have to assume so much responsibility, they frequently use their time to meet the demands of other courses and find themselves far behind in our course. Bargaining sessions frequently ensue in which they try to limit the scope of the examination, delay the final, and so on. I delight in the give and take of the negotiations in which we engage, as it reflects an equality and an authenticity in our relationship. I generally remain tough; if the students are to learn responsibility assumption, they must not be let off the responsibility hook lightly.

My sense of teaching this way is that the students get as much, and often more, content than they did when I took sole responsibility for content. I also am astonished at the interesting byways of content that emerge out of the students' interests. For example, a recent aural rehabilitation class decided to read the play *Children of a Lesser God,* which involves the relationship between a deaf woman and a hearing male speech therapist. From the in-class play reading and discussion, the students obtained a great deal of insight into the problems of deaf–hearing relationships and of contemporary issues among deaf adults. The understanding obtained was of a much deeper dimension than they would have obtained from a review of the didactic literature alone.

Evidence in the literature suggests that locus of control can be shifted to a more internal orientation as a result of learning or teaching experiences. Johnson and Croft (1975) found that students enrolled in a personalized system of instruction (PSI) course demonstrated a statistically significant internally oriented shift as measured by the Rotter scale after the students completed the course. The PSI course has no midterm or final examination; it is entirely self-paced and self-graded. Performance is often evaluated in a personal interview. This sort of course can be modified to become a marvelous blend of behaviorist and humanist notions. Similarly based courses, which would include more contact with the teacher within a humanistic relationship, could be developed within the field of communication disorders in order to develop self-managing students who also have experienced a clinically and personally useful relationship with a teacher.

In these professionally perilous times of high burnout rate and declining student enrollment, we must find creative solutions to implementing humanistic-based education that encourages an inner locus of control. This is not to say that we should give up our cognitive and evaluative functions; we must supplement content with interpersonal learning. It is unreasonable to expect students trained within the current poorly conceived behavioral model to easily take responsibility for themselves and for the profession. The behavioral model, with its emphasis on external locus of control and external locus of evaluation, tends to produce professionals who will accept poor working conditions, work mechanically, and not take responsibility for furthering the profession—by passively and compliantly accepting things as they are. If we do not anticipate change and act, we will be overwhelmed by it. The future of our profession, I think, rests in altering our current educational practices to include a more humanistic base, which will in turn create a more self-confident, self-reliant, and assertive professional, one who will also be much more effective in serving persons with communication disorders. We owe our clients and our profession nothing less.

Professional Burnout

The problem of professional burnout in the helping professions is quite severe. Meadow (1981) administered a burnout inventory to 240 teachers of the deaf. Among the findings of her study were the following:

- Teachers of the deaf had a higher burnout rate than classroom teachers who were teaching children with normal hearing.
- Burnout was highest among teachers who had been working 7 to 10 years in the job and was lowest among teachers who had been working 11 or more years and among new teachers.

- Burnout was directly related to perceived ability to influence the work situation. Teachers who felt they had the power to influence their jobs showed the least burnout.

- Teachers who showed the highest personal involvement in their jobs also tended to have the highest burnout rate.

These results are very interesting. Greater stress appears to occur among professionals working with handicapped populations than among professionals working with nonhandicapped populations. Young teachers seem to be carried through their first years by idealism and enthusiasm. From the Meadow (1981) data and from my own observation, many young beginning teachers get overinvolved with the children. Mattingly (1977) noticed this phenomenon among childcare workers: Burnout was signaled by workers who began to merge themselves and their lives with the institution. When this merging occurs, the individual loses the resources to give to others. A helping professional is very much like a gasoline station where people come to fill up. At some point, a truck comes and fills the tanks of the gasoline station. The professional who merges with the population he or she is serving is always among needy people and has little opportunity to "fill his or her own tank." I think that this is the one who burns out within that 7- to 10-year period.

Those professionals who survive beyond the 10-year period learn better coping strategies probably because they have learned to meet their personal needs outside of their work experiences; from the Meadow (1981) data, it would also seem that they have a more internal locus of control than do the burnout sufferers, since burnout is directly related to the perceived inability to influence the work situation. Teachers with an inner locus of control are not "pushed into" accepting poor working conditions and are also more likely to assert themselves with administrators.

Within the context and terminologies of this book, burnout can be viewed as primarily a problem in dealing with the existential issue of loneliness and love: The need to be loved can push the teacher into an unwholesome, overinvolved relationship with the students. Using the Erikson model, burnout can also be seen as an intimacy issue in that there is a fusion of the personal life and the job. I think that overall burnout is a locus of control problem because people who feel that they have no power, who are like "leaves in the wind" simply meeting other people's demands, will lose all feeling for their clients, will become emotionally exhausted and drained, and will burn out.

I think that we can effect changes in the burnout phenomenon by providing ongoing workshops and inservice training for working professionals. I think that a more efficient way of dealing with this problem is by producing students who value themselves, who have an awareness of their own needs, who have an ability to be authentic in relationships, and who have a more internal locus of control and locus of evaluation.

Counseling Within the Public Schools

The public school setting is a difficult milieu for counseling to occur. The typical therapy model for the public school setting is one in which the children are taken out of class for individual therapy. Because of caseload numbers, therapists sometimes offer therapy in small groups. Contact with the parents is usually minimal, very often just a phone call, more often simply messages carried back and forth by the child. It has always struck me that the underlying assumptions of this therapy model are incredibly naive. It assumes in effect that by working in isolation with the child for one hour a week (in some cases for only half an hour), a therapist can significantly alter the child's communication skills. It presupposes an incredibly powerful effect of individual therapy. It also burdens the child to be the change agent for the whole family system.

I think many therapists in the public schools intuitively recognize the absurdity of their professional lives. The restrictions they have accepted, either because those restrictions have been externally imposed or because of an internal reluctance to risk changing them, do not allow the therapists to do an effective job. When that happens, they either leave their jobs quickly or they burn out and go through the motions of the job knowing full well that they are being ineffective.

I think there are ways to restructure jobs so that therapists become effective change agents. Therapists need to see themselves as consultants/counselors rather than as direct purveyors of therapy. Therapy, where possible, needs to be directed at the parents in order to be more effective. Within the public school setting, the teachers have the parental role. We can be much more efficient if we alter the classroom environment, which is the child's home away from home, so that it becomes more facilitative for the development of good communication skills for all the children. This means we must spend our time with the teachers in the classroom, helping them to help the children with communication disorders.

I think this consultative model of speech pathology is slowly taking hold and will become the dominant therapeutic model of the 1990s. Superior and Leichook (1986) strongly recommended a parent consultant model within the public school setting. They suggested that "parent meetings could be scheduled in lieu of the child's treatment sessions providing that the goal of parent consultation be addressed within the individual education plan. A few parent meetings may, in fact, have far greater effect than several therapy sessions" (p. 402). My sense is that the time spent with parents or teachers is usually the most fruitful time, and the thrust of therapy needs to be at the teacher/parent level.

In setting up the consultation model, it is critical that the therapist, before initiating any direct therapy with the child, meet with the classroom teachers and the child's parents. At this time a clear contract needs to be drawn up that specifies the expectations of everyone. I think the therapist needs to move toward a contract with the parents and the teachers that requires them to have some direct involvement in the therapeutic process. The contract has to be flexible and opportunities must be provided for renegotiation. If there is any failure to meet contractual expectations, then the teacher/parent has to be called on the carpet. It is absolutely essential that a working relationship be established before the initiation of therapy. This establishes the basis for any ongoing disputes involving the child directly or the contractual obligations.

The major area where parents and therapists interact is around developing the Individualized Educational Plan (IEP) for the child. In poorly run programs, the process is usually painful for the parents as they are subjected to the reports of the professionals in an arena style conference. Parents usually leave intimidated and more confused than they went into the confusion; certainly not empowered. Andrews and Andrews (1993) have presented a model of developing an educational plan that serves to empower parents, and I think this model needs to be adopted widely. In the Andrews' approach, which is very family centered, all members of the family are encouraged to participate. The families are listened to and encouraged to participate actively in the assessment of the child. The authors present enabling techniques adapted from family therapy approaches that are readily within the grasp of professionals who work with persons with communication disorders.

Multiculturalism

In a fascinating article, Van Kleeck (1994) has described the many cultural traps that the insensitive speech–language pathologist can fall into. For example, when the speech–language pathologist assumes that getting the child to initiate more communication means getting the child to initiate conversation with adults, he or she may be unwittingly violating a family norm. In many cultures, children are not encouraged to initiate conversations with adults. The danger is ever present that we impose our cultural values on others. It is so easy to operate from our own ethnocentric perspective that we fail to appreciate cultural differences.

On the other hand, there is an equal danger that in looking for cultural differences among populations, we fall into the trap of cultural stereotyping.

Within any cultural grouping, there are always variations in behavior, and the generalizations we might make about a population may not apply to the specific individual with whom we are working. What needs to be understood is that in one sense we are all multicultural; each family must be approached as a marvelous experiment of one. We must take each family as they come and allow them to teach us the best way for them to learn. We always need to respect the dignity of each family we encounter, and, as Van Kleeck (1994) has pointed out, we must create an educational program to fit the family rather than try to fit the family to our program. This notion undergirds everything that is in this text. By listening to and valuing our clients, we will always respect their unique cultural heritage.

The Limits of Counseling

In a thoughtful article, Stone and Olswang (1989) tried to define the boundaries for counseling by speech pathologists and audiologists. They argued that many times the problem is not that we need better counseling skills, but that the client should be referred to a mental health professional. The boundary for this referral is very hard to define, and Stone and Olswang failed to offer clear guidelines. I am not sure I have any clear guidelines either. I have found that as I become more comfortable with myself and more comfortable with affect in my relationships, my professional boundaries have expanded and I am willing to allow my professional relationships much greater latitude. I find myself less willing to refer clients. It is very difficult to refer a client to a mental health professional in such a way that does not provoke extreme anxiety in the client. The message you are sending to the client, no matter how nicely put, is that the problem is so formidable that he or she needs to see someone else. This is often very threatening to clients.

In actuality, the person with the problem in that situation is often the speech pathologist or audiologist. I think psychologists and social workers who are employed in clinics need to provide ongoing inservice training to the speech pathologists/audiologists to help them increase their counseling skills and confidence in their ability to relate on the affect level with clients. This requires the mental health professional to be professionally secure and able to accept a consultative role. Unfortunately, there are many "Annie Sullivan" psychologists and social workers who are anxious to rescue the speech pathologist/audiologist; this "de-skills" them in the same way that Annie de-skilled Mrs. Keller.

Undoubtedly, there are people with emotional disturbance who develop communication disorders or who are the relatives of someone with a communication disorder. These people are not normally upset, although they may seem so at the beginning, but are truly emotionally disturbed individuals with a multitude of life adjustment problems. I have a responsibility to identify these clients and then to set my limits. I do not refer clients to mental health professionals because I don't presume to know what is best for someone else. I have clear boundaries for myself, and I will tell clients that I do not feel professionally comfortable and do not want to delve further. Clients then generally refer themselves for further counseling. If they ask me for a referral, I am able to give them the names of two or three people to consult; I won't make the choice for them.

Counseling skills permeate everything I do. I do not want us or expect us as a profession to charge for "counseling." This is something a mental health professional does and it would be an inappropriate professional invasion. What we need to be doing is infusing counseling notions in everything we do. Many of the problems we encounter with clients can be solved by using techniques culled from the family therapy literature. Stone (1992) has demonstrated how a systems approach can be used to analyze problematic relationships so as to improve the interactions between the professional and the families involved in the therapy. As mentioned previously, Andrews and Andrews (1993) used system theory to help empower families during the IEP process. I think this trend will continue as we discover and utilize material and techniques garnered from the psychotherapy literature.

I think the key to counseling is the congruence of the counselor. As I become more congruent, technique slips away or, more accurately, becomes incorporated into everything I do. I think the most important thing a counselor brings to the helping relationship is self. The importance of the congruent professional far exceeds the value of any diagnostic test or specific techniques in counseling. If the literature on the desirable personality characteristics of the counselor were examined, it would appear that no one would qualify unless one could also qualify for sainthood. It is not necessary to be an entirely self-actualized person to be an effective counselor; rather, I think one needs to have a deep interest in people and a sensitivity to others. One needs to be a caring individual who does not impose beliefs on others, who maintains a constant awareness of self, and who does not hide behind the artificiality of being a professional. Our growth as a profession will be measured by how we grow as individuals. We owe our profession and our clients our commitment to learn about ourselves as well as our field; we can do no less.

References

Albertini, J., Smith, J., & Metz, D. (1983). Small group versus individual speech therapy with hearing impaired young adults. *Volta Review, 85,* 83–87.

Alpiner, J. (1978). Ancillary personnel in rehabilitation. In S. Alpiner (Ed.), *Handbook of adult rehabilitative audiology* (pp. 232–274). Baltimore: Williams & Wilkins.

Andrews, M. A. (1986). Application of family therapy techniques to the treatment of language disorders. *Seminars in Speech and Language, 7,* 347–358.

Andrews, M., & Andrews, J. (1993). Family-centered techniques: Integrating enablement into the IFSP process. *Journal of Childhood Communication Disorders, 15*(1), 41–46.

Arbuckle, D. S. (1970). *Counseling: Philosophy, theory and practice* (2nd ed.). Boston: Allyn & Bacon.

Asha Interview: Geri Jewell. (1983). *Asha, 25,* 18–22.

Atkins, D. (Ed.). (1987). Families and their hearing impaired children. *Volta Review, 89* (Monograph No. 5).

Backus, O., & Beasley, J. (1951). *Speech therapy with children.* Cambridge, MA: Houghton Mifflin.

Bardach, J. (1969). Group sessions with wives of aphasic patients. *International Journal of Group Psychotherapy, 119,* 361–366.

Baumgarten, M., Battista, R., Infante-Rivard, M., Hanley, J., Becker, R., & Gauthier, S. (1990). The psychological and physical health of family members caring for an elderly person with dementia. *Journal of Clinical Epidemiology, 45*(1), 61–70.

Beavers, R., & Voeller, M. (1983). Comparing and contrasting the Olson Circumplex Model with the Beavers Systems Model. *Family Process, 22,* 85–98.

Berry, J. O. (1987). Strategies for involving parents for young children using augmentative and alternative communication. *Augmentative and Alternative Communication, 3*(2), 90–93.

Bodner, B., & Johns, J. (1977). Personality and hearing impairment: A study in locus of control. *Volta Review, 79,* 362–368.

Bynner, W. (Trans.). (1962). *The way of life according to Lao-tze.* New York: Capricorn Books.

Caracciolo, G., Rigrodsky, S., & Morrison, E. (1978). A Rogerian orientation to the speech–language pathology supervisory relationship. *Asha, 20,* 286–290.

Cartwright, L., & Ruscello, D. (1979). A survey on parent involvement in speech clinics. *Asha, 21,* 275–280.

Cole, S., O'Conner, S., & Bennett, L. (1979). Self-help groups for clinic patients with chronic illness. *Primary Care, 6*(2), 325–339.

Coles, R. (1970). *Erik H. Erikson: The growth of his work.* Boston: Little, Brown.

Cook, J. (1964). Silences in psychotherapy. *Journal of Counseling Psychology, 11,* 42–46.

Cooper, E. (1966). Client–clinician relationships and concomitant factors in stuttering therapy. *Journal of Speech and Hearing Disorders, 9,* 194–199.

Cottrel, A., Montague, J., Farb, J., & Throne, S. (1980). An operant procedure for improving vocabulary definition performance in developmentally delayed children. *Journal of Speech and Hearing Disorders, 45,* 90–95.

Craig, A., Franklin, J., & Andrews, G. (1985). The prediction and prevention of relapse in stuttering. *Behavior Modification, 9,* 422–442.

Crane, S., & Cooper, E. (1983). Speech–language clinician personality variables and clinical effectiveness. *Journal of Speech and Hearing Disorders, 48,* 140–147.

Crowley, M., Keane, K., & Needham, C. (1982). Fathers: The forgotten parents. *American Annals of the Deaf, 127,* 38–45.

Culatta, R., Colucci, S., & Wiggins, E. (1975). Clinical supervisors and trainees: Two views of a process. *Asha, 171,* 152–156.

Culpepper, B., Mendel, L., & McCarthy, P. (1994). Counseling experience and training offered by ESB-accredited programs. *ASHA, 36,* 55–64.

Dale, P. (1991). The validity of a parent report measure of vocabulary and syntax at 24 months. *Journal of Speech and Hearing Research, 34,* 565–571.

Darius, B. (1988). *A study of siblings of hearing impaired children: How they were affected by the handicap.* Unpublished master's thesis, Emerson College, Boston.

Davies, H., Priddy, M., & Tinkleberg, J. (1986). Support groups for male caregivers of Alzheimer's patients. *Clinical Gerontologist, 5,* 385–394.

Dee, A. (1981). Meeting the needs of the parents of deaf infants. *Language, Speech and Hearing Services in Schools, 12,* 13–21.

Dowaliby, F., Burke, N., & McKee, B. (1983). A comparison of hearing impaired and normally hearing students on locus of control, people orientation and study habits and attitudes. *American Annals of the Deaf, 128,* 53–59.

Dundon, M., Carmer, S., & Novak, C. (1987). *Distress and coping among caregivers of victims of Alzheimer's disease.* Paper presented at the annual meeting of the American Psychological Association, New York.

Edgerly, R. (1975). *The effectiveness of parent counseling in the treatment of children with learning disabilities.* Unpublished doctoral dissertation, Boston University.

Egolf, D., Shames, G., Johnson, P., & Kasprisin-Burrell, S. (1972). The use of parent interaction patterns in therapy for young stutterers. *Journal of Speech and Hearing Disorders, 37,* 222–227.

Ellis, A. (1977). The basic clinical theory of rational–emotive therapy. In A. Ellis & R. Grieger (Eds.), *Handbook of rational–emotive therapy* (pp. 11–19). New York: Springer.

Emerick, L. (1988). Counseling adults who stutter: A cognitive approach. *Seminars in Speech and Language, 9,* 257–267.

Emerson, R. (1980). *Changes in depression and self-esteem of spouses of stroke patients with aphasia as a result of group counseling.* Unpublished doctoral dissertation, Oregon University, Eugene.

Epstein, N., Bishop, D., & Baldwin, L. (1982). McMaster model of family functioning: A view of the normal family. In F. Walsh (Ed.), *Normal family process* (pp. 148–172). New York: Guilford Press.

Erikson, E. H. (1950). *Childhood and society* (2nd ed.). New York: Norton.

Farran, C., Keane-Hagerty, E., Salloway, S., Kupferer, S., & Wilken, C. (1991). Finding meaning: An alternative paradigm for Alzheimer's disease family caregivers. *The Gerontologist, 31*(4), 483–489.

Featherstone, H. (1980). *A difference in the family.* New York: Basic Books.

Flahive, M., & White, S. (1982). Audiologists and counseling. *Journal of the Academy of Rehabilitative Audiology, 10,* 275–287.

Fleming, M. (1972). A total approach to communication therapy. *Journal of the Academy of Rehabilitative Audiology, 5,* 28–35.

Fromm, E. (1941). *Escape from freedom.* New York: Holt, Rinehart & Winston.

Gallagher, J. J., Cross, A., & Scharfman, W. (1981). Parental adaptation to a young handicapped child: The father's role. *Journal of the Division for Early Childhood, 3,* 3–14.

Gardner, H. (1991). *The unschooled mind.* New York: Basic Books.

Gath, A. (1977). The impact of the abnormal child upon the parents. *British Society of Psychiatry, 130,* 405–410.

Girolametta, M. E., Greenberg, J., & Manolson, A. (1986). Developing dialogue skills: The Hanen early language parent program. *Seminars in Speech and Language, 7,* 367–382.

Gregory, H. (1983). *The clinician's attitudes in counseling stutterers* (Publication No. 18). Memphis: Speech Foundation of America.

Grossman, F. K. (1972). *Brothers and sisters of retarded children.* Syracuse: Syracuse University Press.

Haas, W. H., & Crowley, D. S. (1982). Professional information dissemination to parents of preschool hearing-impaired children. *Volta Review, 84,* 17–23.

Hallahan, P., Gasar, A., Cohen, S., & Tarver, S. (1978). Selective attention and locus of control in learning disabled and normal children. *Journal of the Learning Disabled, 11,* 47–57.

Hansen, J., Stavis, R., & Warner, R. (1977). *Counseling theory and process.* Boston: Allyn & Bacon.

Harris, S., Handiman, J., & Palmer, C. (1985). Parents and grandparents view the autistic child. *Journal of Autism and Developmental Disorders, 15,* 125–135.

Harvey, M. (1989). *Psychotherapy with deaf and hard of hearing persons: A systemic model.* Hillsdale, NJ: Erlbaum.

Hinkle, S. (1991). Support group counseling for the caregivers of Alzheimer's disease patients. *The Journal for Specialists in Group Work, 16*(3), 185–190.

Hoffman, L. (1981). *Foundations of family therapy.* New York: Basic Books.

Holt, J. (1964). *How children fail.* New York: Dell.

Hornyak, A. (1980). The rescue game and the speech–language pathologist. *Asha, 22,* 86–94.

Israelite, N. K. (1986). Hearing impaired children and the psychological functioning of their normal hearing siblings. *Volta Review, 88,* 47–54.

Johnson, W., & Croft, R. (1975). Locus of control and participation in a personalized system of instruction course. *Journal of Educational Psychology, 67,* 416–421.

Kazak, A., & Marvin, R. (1984). Differences, difficulties and adaptations: Stress and social networks in families with a handicapped child. *Family Relationships, 33,* 67–77.

Klevans, D., Volz, H., & Friedman, R. (1981). A comparison of experimental and observational approaches for enhancing the interpersonal communication skills of speech–language pathology students. *Journal of Speech and Hearing Disorders, 46,* 208–212.

Kommers, M. S., & Sullivan, M. D. (1979). Wives' evaluation of problems related to laryngectomy. *Journal of Communicative Disorders, 12,* 411–418.

Kopp, S. (1972). *If you meet the Buddha on the road kill him!* Palo Alto: Science and Behavioral Books.

Kopp, S. (1978). *An end to innocence.* New York: Bantam.

Kornhaber, C., & Woodward, L. (1985). *Grandparents/grandchildren—The vital connection.* New Brunswick, NJ: Transaction Books.

Kubler-Ross, E. (1969). *On death and dying.* New York: Macmillan.

Land, S. L., & Vineberg, S. E. (1965). Locus of control in blind children. *Exceptional Child, 31,* 257–263.

Lash, J. V. (1980). *Helen and teacher.* New York: Delacorte.

Lavell, N., & Keogh, B. (1980). Expectation and attribution of parents of handicapped children. In S. S. Gallagher (Ed.), *Parents and families of handicapped children* (pp. 48–72). San Francisco: Jossey-Bass.

Lear, M. (1980). *Heartsounds.* New York: Simon & Schuster.

Lerner, W. (1988). *Parents' and audiologists' perspectives regarding counseling.* Unpublished master's thesis, Emerson College, Boston.

Levine, S. (1979). *A gradual awakening.* New York: Anchor.

Levine, S. (1982). *Who dies.* New York: Anchor.

Lieberman, M., Yalom, I., & Miles, M. (1973). *Encounter groups: First facts.* New York: Basic Books.

Lloyd, L., Spradlin, J., & Reid, M. (1968). An operant audiometric procedure for difficult-to-test patients. *Journal of Speech and Hearing Disorders, 33,* 236–242.

Lobato, D. (1983). Siblings of handicapped children: A review. *Journal of Autism and Developmental Disabilities, 13,* 347–364.

Lowe, T. (1989). *Grandparents view the hearing impaired child.* Unpublished master's thesis, Emerson College, Boston.

Lund, N. J. (1986). Family events and relationships: Implications for language assessment and intervention. *Seminars in Speech and Language, 7,* 415–436.

Luterman, D. (1969). Hypothetical families. *Volta Review, 71,* 347–351.

Luterman, D. (1979). *Counseling parents of hearing impaired children.* Boston: Little, Brown.

Luterman, D. (1987). *Deafness in the family.* Boston: Little, Brown.

Luterman, D. (1995). *In the shadows: Living and coping with a loved one's chronic illness.* Bedford, MA: Jade Press.

Madison, L., Budd, K., & Itzkowitz, J. (1986). Changes in stuttering in relation to children's locus of control. *Journal of Genetic Psychology, 147,* 233–240.

Malone, R. L. (1969). Expressed attitudes of families of aphasics. *Journal of Speech and Hearing Disorders, 34,* 146–151.

Martin, F., George, K., O'Neal, J., & Daly, J. (1987). Audiologists' and parents' attitudes regarding counseling of families of hearing impaired children. *Asha, 29,* 27–33.

Martin, F., Krueger, S., & Bernstein, M. (1990). Diagnostic information transfer to hearing-impaired adults. *Texas Journal of Audiology and Speech Pathology, 16*(2), 29–32.

Maslow, A. H. (1962). *Towards a psychology of being.* Trenton, NJ: Van Nordstrand.

Massie, R., & Massie, S. (1973). *Journey.* New York: Knopf.

Matis, E. (1961). Psychotherapeutic tools for parents. *Journal of Speech and Hearing Disorders, 26,* 164–170.

Matson, D., & Brooks, L. (1977). Adjusting to multiple sclerosis: An explorative study. *Social Science and Medicine, 11,* 245–250.

Mattingly, M. A. (1977). Sources of stress and burnout in professional child care work. *Child Care Quarterly, 6,* 127–130.

Maxwell, D. (1982). Cognitive and behavioral self-control strategies: Applications for the clinical management of adult stutterers. *Journal of Fluency Disorders, 7,* 403–432.

McCarthy, P., Culpepper, N., & Lucks, L. (1986). Variability in counseling experiences and training among ESB accredited programs. *Asha, 28,* 49–53.

McKelvey, J., & Borgersen, M. (1990). Family development and the use of diabetes groups: Experience with a model approach. *Patient Education and Counseling, 16,* 61–67.

Meadow, K. (1981). Burnout in professionals working with deaf children. *American Annals of the Deaf, 126,* 13–19.

Mendelsohn, M., & Rozek, F. (1983). Denying disability: The case of deafness. *Family Systems Medicine, 1*(2), 37–47.

Miller, M., & Potter, R. (1982). Professional burnout among speech–language pathologists. *Asha, 24,* 177–180.

Minuchin, S. (1974). *Families and family therapy.* Cambridge, MA: Harvard University Press.

Minuchin, S., Rosman, B., & Baker, L. (1978). *Psychosomatic families.* Cambridge, MA: Harvard University Press.

Mitford, J. (1963). *The American way of death.* New York: Simon & Schuster.

Moore, P. (1982). Voice disorders. In G. Shames & E. Wiig (Eds.), *Human communication disorders* (pp. 312–346). Columbus, OH: Merrill.

Moustakes, C. (1961). *Loneliness.* Englewood Cliffs, NJ: Prentice-Hall.

Munro, J., & Bach, T. (1975). Effect of time limited counseling on client change. *Journal of Counseling Psychology, 22,* 395–406.

Murphy, A. (1981). *Special children, special parents.* Englewood Cliffs, NJ: Prentice-Hall.

Murphy, A. (1982). The clinical process and the speech–language pathologist. In G. Shames & E. Wiig (Eds.), *Human communication disorders* (pp. 386–402). Columbus, OH: Merrill.

Nuland, S.D. (1994). *How we die.* New York: Knopf.

Olson, D., Russell, C., & Sprenkle, D. (1983). Circumflex model of marital and family systems: VI. Theoretical update. *Family Process, 22,* 69–83.

Pearlin, L., & Schooler, S. (1978). The structure of coping. *Journal of Health and Social Behavior, 19,* 2–21.

Peck, S. (1978). *The road less traveled.* New York: Simon & Schuster.

Pedersen, F. (1976). Does research on children reared in father absent families yield information on father influences? *Family Coordinator, 25,* 459–463.

Perkins, W. P. (1977). *Speech pathology: An applied behavioral science* (2nd ed.). St. Louis: Mosby.

Pickering, M. (1977). An examination of concepts operative in the supervisory process and relationship. *Asha, 19,* 697–770.

Post, J. (1983). I'd rather tell a story than be one. *Asha, 25,* 22–25.

Rabins, P. (1984). Management of dementia in the family context. *Psychosomatics, 25,* 369–375.

Rimm, D. C., & Cunningham, H. M. (1985). Behavior therapies. In S. J. Lynn & J. P. Garske (Eds.), *Contemporary psychotherapies* (pp. 44–70). Columbus, OH: Merrill.

Robertson, E., & Suinn, R. (1968). The determination of rate of progress of stroke patients through empathy measures of patient and family. *Journal of Psychosomatic Research, 12,* 189–193.

Rogers, C. (1951). *Client centered therapy.* Boston: Houghton Mifflin.

Rogers, C. (1980). *A way of being.* Boston: Houghton Mifflin.

Rollins, W. (1988). Counseling spouses of the communicatively impaired. *Seminars in Speech and Language, 9,* 269–277.

Rotter, S. (1966). Generalized expectancies for internal versus external control of reinforcement. *Psychology Monographs: General and Applied, 1* (Whole No. 609).

Roy, R. (1990). Consequences of parental illness on children: A review. *Social Work and Social Sciences Review, 2*(2), 109–121.

Sabbeth, B., & Leventhal, J. (1988). Trial balloons: When families of ill children express needs in veiled ways. *Children's Health Care, 171,* 87–92.

Sager, C. (1978). *Marriage contract and couple therapy.* New York: Rawson, Wade.

Sandow, S., & Clarke, D. B. (1977). Home intervention with parents of severely subnormal, preschool children: An interim report. *Child Care, Health and Development, 4,* 29–39.

Satir, V. (1967). *Conjoint family therapy.* Palo Alto, CA: Science & Behavior Books.

Schein, J. (1982). Group techniques applied to deaf and hearing-impaired persons. In M. Seligman (Ed.), *Group psychotherapy and counseling with special populations* (pp. 41–60). Baltimore: University Park Press.

Schlessinger, H., & Meadow, K. (1971). *Deafness and mental health: A developmental approach* (Report No. RD283-S). Washington, DC: U.S. Department of Health, Education, and Welfare.

Schlessinger, H. (1994). The elusive X factor: Parental contributions to literacy. In M. Walworth, D. Moones, & T. O'Rourke (Eds.), *A free hand* (pp. 37–66). Silver Springs, MD: TS Publishers.

Schwirian, P. (1976). Effects of the presence of a hearing impaired preschool child in the family on behavior patterns of older "normal" siblings. *American Annals of the Deaf, 121,* 373–380.

Seligman, M. (1982). *Group psychotherapy and counseling with special populations.* Baltimore: University Park Press.

Seligman, M., & Lobato, D. (1983). Siblings of handicapped persons. In M. Seligman (Ed.), *The family with a handicapped child: Understanding and treatment* (pp. 3–27). New York: Grune & Stratton.

Shames, G., & Florance, C. (1982). Disorders of fluency. In G. Shames & E. Wag (Eds.), *Human communication disorders* (pp. 86–110). Columbus, OH: Merrill.

Shirlberg, L., Diabless, D., Carlson, K., Filley, F., Kwiatkowski, J., & Smith, M. (1977). Personality characteristics, academic performance and clinical competence in communication disorders majors. *Asha, 19,* 311–315.

Shlien, J., Mosak, H., & Dreikors, R. (1962). Effects of time limits: A comparison of the psychotherapies. *Journal of Counseling Psychology, 9,* 31–36.

Singler, J. (1982). The stroke group: Planning for success. In M. Seligman (Ed.), *Group psychotherapy and counseling with special populations* (pp. 170–196). Baltimore: University Park Press.

Ski Hi, Communicative Disorders Institute. (1985). [National Summer Conference]. Utah State University, Ogden.

Skinner, B. F. (1953). *Science and human behavior.* New York: Macmillan.

Starkweather, C. (1974). Behavior modification in training speech clinicians: Procedures and implications. *Asha, 16,* 607–612.

Stech, E., Curtiss, J., Troesch, P., & Binnie, C. (1973). Clients' reinforcement of speech clinicians: A factor analytic study. *Asha, 15,* 287–291.

Stone, J. (1992). Resolving relationship problems in communication disorders treatment: A systems approach. *Language, Speech and Hearing Services in Schools, 23,* 300–307.

Stone, J. R., & Olswang, L. B. (1989). The hidden challenge in counseling. *Asha, 31,* 27–30.

Superior, K., & Leichook, A. (1986). Family participation in school based programs. *Seminars in Speech and Language, 7,* 395–414.

Tanner, D. C. (1980). Loss and grief implications for the speech–language pathologist and audiologist. *Asha, 22,* 916–922.

VanKleeck, A. (1994). Potential cultural bias in training parents as conversational partners with their children who have delays in language development. *ASHA, 35,* 67–76.

Van Riper, C. (1965). Supervision of clinical practice. *Asha, 7,* 75–78.

Venters, M. (1981). Familial coping with chronic and severe childhood illness: The case of cystic fibrosis. *Social Science and Medicine, 15A,* 289–297.

Ventimiglia, R. (1986). Helping couples with neurological disabilities: A job description for clinical sociologists. *Clinical Sociology Review, 4,* 123–139.

Ward, B., & Webster, E. (1965). The training of clinical personnel: A concept of clinical preparation. *Asha, 7,* 103–108.

Webster, E. (1966). Parent counseling by speech pathologists and audiologists. *Journal of Speech and Hearing Disorders, 31,* 331–345.

Webster, E. (1968). Procedures for group counseling in speech pathology and audiology. *Journal of Speech and Hearing Disorders, 33,* 27–35.

Webster, E. (1977). *Counseling with parents of handicapped children.* New York: Grune & Stratton.

Webster, M. (1982). *Hear Here Newsletter of the Canadian Speech and Hearing, 6,* 235–237.

White, K. (1982). Defining and prioritizing the personal and social competence needed by hearing impaired students. *Volta Review, 84,* 266–273.

Williams, D. M. L., & Derbyshire, J. O. (1982). Diagnosis of deafness: A study of family responses and needs. *Volta Review, 84,* 24–30.

Wright, D. (1969). *Deafness.* New York: Stein & Day.

Yalom, I. (1975). *The theory and practice of group psychotherapy.* New York: Basic Books.

Yalom, I. (1980). *Existential psychotherapy.* New York: Basic Books.

Yalom, I. (1989). *Love's executioner.* New York: Basic Books.

Yarnell, G. (1983). Comparisons of operant and conventional audiometric procedures with multihandicapped (deaf-blind) children. *Volta Review, 85,* 69–74.

Index

Acceptance stage of coping process, 70
Addictions, 18
Adolescence, 147–148
Affect. *See* Emotions
Affect release, through group process,
        116–117
Affect response, as counseling technique,
        91–92
Affirmation, as counseling technique,
        94–95
Affirmation stage, in coping process,
        69–70
ALS, 92
Altruism, through group process, 114
Alzheimer's disease, 20, 112, 150, 163
Amyotrophic lateral sclerosis (ALS), 92
Anger, 53–57, 63, 143
Aphasia, 112, 135
Audiologists. *See also* Professionals
    boundaries for counseling by, 177–178
    counseling by, 1–7
    ineffectiveness of, in counseling, 2–3
    training in counseling for, 2, 167–173
Autism, 152
Autonomy
    autonomy versus shame and doubt in
        Erikson life cycle, 32–33,36
    in counseling relationship, 39–40

Behavior modification, 11–12
Behavioral counseling
    for communication disorders, 11–12
    compared with other counseling
        theories, 28
    contracting in, 104–105
    description of, 10–11
    limitations of, 12–13

Brain damage, 22, 164
Burnout, 169, 173–175

Catharsis, through group process, 115
Cause of disorder, 84
Cerebral palsy, 162
Changing-topic silence, 103–104
Childhood and Society, 31
Children of a Lesser God, 172
Chronic illness, 66, 112, 136–139, 149
Client-centered counseling, 13–14
Client-centered diagnosis, 77–85
Client Centered Therapy (Rogers), 13
Client versus patient, 43
Cognitive therapy
    for communication disorders, 26–27
    compared with other counseling
        theories, 28–29
    description of, 25–26
    language changing, 101–102
    limitations of, 27–28
Cohesiveness of groups, 114–115, 126
Conflict
    in families, 160
    in groups, 126, 127
Confrontation norm, 120–121,
        124–125
Confusion feelings, 61–62
Congruence
    of client, 6–7
    of counselor, 14, 178
Consultative model of speech pathology,
        175–176
Content mandate, of group process, 116,
        126–127
Content response, by counselor, 89
Contracting, 104–105

Coping process
   affirmation stage in, 69–70
   definition of coping, 70–71
   denial stage in, 66–68, 77–78, 80,
      143–144, 152, 162
   flight as coping strategy, 71–72
   integration stage of, 70
   modification as coping strategy, 72
   reframing as coping strategy, 72
   resistance stage in, 68–69
   stress reduction as coping strategy, 73
Counseling. *See also* Counseling
   techniques
   author's initial training in, 1
   autonomy in, 39–40
   behavioral counseling, 10–13, 28
   cognitive therapy, 25–28
   compared with parable on blind men
      and elephant, 9
   comparison of theories of, 28–29
   and congruence of client, 6–7
   and congruence of counselor, 14, 178
   effectiveness of, 106–107
   Erikson life cycle and relationship
      building in, 37–46
   existentialism and, 16–24, 28
   generativity in, 45
   humanistic counseling, 13–15, 28
   identity in, 43–44
   by informing, 1–3, 61–62
   initiative in, 40–41
   integrated approach to, 87–88
   integrity in, 45–46
   intimacy in, 44–45
   lack of training in, for speech
      pathologists and audiologists, 2
   limits of, 177–178
   by listening and valuing, 5–7, 109–110
   medical model of, 1–2
   and models as clinical tools, 46
   multiculturalism and, 85, 90, 176–177
   by persuading, 3–5, 27–28
   within public schools, 175–177
   by speech pathologist and audiologist,
      1–7
   training in, 1, 64–65

Counseling techniques. *See also* Group
   process
   affect response, 91–92
   affirmation, 94–95
   case studies of hypothetical families,
      95–99
   cautions about, 87–88
   changing-topic silence, 103–104
   content response, 89
   contracting, 104–105
   counselor control via response, 88–95
   counselor feedback, 105–110
   counterquestions, 90–91
   embarrassed silence, 103
   locus of control, 99–102
   as not bound to particular philosophy,
      88
   reflective silence, 104
   reframing, 92–93
   and sample client questions, 94–95
   sharing self, 93–94
   silence, 102–104
   termination silence, 104
   "uh huh" response, 94
Counselors. *See* Professionals
Counterquestions, as counseling
   technique, 90–91
Credibility establishment, 38
Cultural stereotypes, 176–177

Deafness. *See* Hearing impairments
Deafness in the Family (Luterman), 156
Death
   and existentialism, 16–17, 20–21
   of parent, 150–151
Death fantasies, as coping strategy, 71–72
Dementia, 149–150
Demonstration, 41–42
Denial stage of coping process, 66–68,
      77–78, 80, 143–144, 152, 162
Despair, ego integrity versus, 35
Developmental delay, 12, 154–155
Diagnostic process
   and cause of disorder, 84
   client-centered diagnosis, 77–85
   diagnosis by committee, 76–77

feelings of parents during, 79, 81–83, 85

importance of, 75

individual medical model of, 75–76

information for parents about, 80–81

institution-centered diagnosis, 75–77

medical model of, 75–77

parental involvement in, 77–85

parental self-report in, 78–79

poem about, 81–83

questions of parents during, 80–81, 83–84

reframing during, 83–84

steps in client-centered diagnosis, 85

Disorder, cause of, 84

Divorce, 71

Doing, in learning, 42–43

Doubt and shame, autonomy versus, 32–33, 36

Down's syndrome, 142, 162

Education. *See* Training

Effectiveness of counseling, 106–107

Ego integrity. *See* Integrity

Embarrassed silence, 103

Emotional disturbance, 177–178

Emotions

acknowledgement and acceptance of, 48

affect response as counseling technique, 91–92

anger, 53–57, 63, 143

avoidance of, 47–48

communication of, by men, 143–144

confusion feelings, 61–62

coping process, 66–73

of grandparents, 153

grief, 36, 48–50, 81, 144

guilt, 57–59, 63, 143, 153

inadequacy feelings, 50–53

painful emotions in counseling, 106–107

of parents during diagnostic process, 79, 81–83, 85

of professionals, 62–64, 105–106

release of, through group process, 116–117

training students for parent programs, 64–65

vulnerability feelings, 59–60, 63

Empathic listening, 14, 91

Empowerment of families, 161–162

Erikson life cycle

autonomy versus shame and doubt, 32–33, 36

communication disorders and, 35–37

ego integrity versus despair, 35

and Erikson's life, 31

generativity versus stagnation, 35

identity versus role confusion, 33–34

industry versus inferiority, 33, 36

initiative versus guilt, 33, 36

intimacy versus isolation, 34–35

model of, as clinical tool, 46

and relationship building in counseling, 37–46

stages of, 32–35

trust versus mistrust, 32, 36

undelying assumptions of, 32

Escape from Freedom (Fromm), 18

Existentialism

applied to communication disorders, 20–24

compared with other counseling models, 28

death and, 16–17, 20–21

description of, 16–20

group process and, 116

limitations of, 24

loneliness and, 19, 22–23

meaninglessness and, 20, 23–24

model of, as clinical tool, 46

responsibility and, 17–19, 21–22

Expectations

in counseling relationship, 55–56

of deaf population as low achievers, 21, 36

violation of parents' expectations over disability of child, 53–54

External locus of control, 100–102

Families. *See also* Parents

children of disability in, 147–151

components of, 136–159
empowerment of, 161–162
grandparents in, 151–154, 164
importance of, 131–132
optimal families, 159–161
parents in, 139–147
shared burden in, 163
siblings in, 154–159
spouses in, 136–139
stress on, 146–147, 164–165
successful families, 161–165
as system, 133
triangulation in, 140–141
Family therapy, 132–136
Fathers, 140–142, 145–146
Feedback by counselor
on counselor's feelings about client,
105–106
and effectiveness of counseling, 106–107
mistakes by counselor, 108–109
professional humility, 107–108
and unattractive client, 109
Feelings. *See* Emotions
Flight as coping strategy, 71–72

Generativity
in counseling relationship, 45
generativity versus stagnation in
Erikson life cycle, 35
Grandparents, 151–154, 164
Grief, 36, 48–50, 81, 144
Group norms, 118–123
Group process
affect release through, 116–117
altruism through, 114
catharsis through, 115
cohesiveness in, 114–115, 126
conflict and, 126, 127
content mandate of, 116, 126–127
curative factors in groups, 113–16
existential issues in, 116
filling available time, 130
and goals in communication disorders,
116–117
group norms established, 118–123
homogeneity of grouping, 128–129
hope instilled through, 113

inception of group, 123–126
information imparted through, 113–114
interpersonal learning through, 114
leadership in, 117–118
personal growth through, 117
principles of group functioning,
117–123
resistance to, 125–126
size and setting of group, 129–130
in speech pathology and audiology,
111–113
stages of group development, 123–127
structured experiences and, 128
terminating group, 127
trust and, 127
universality of feelings recognized
through, 113
working group, 126–127
Group psychotherapy, 112–113
Guilt
initiative versus guilt in Erikson life
cycle, 33, 36
of parents, 57–59, 143, 153
of professionals, 63

Hearing impairments, 22, 35–36, 112,
135–136, 156–158, 164
Heartsounds (Lear), 43
Hemophilia, 23
Here-and-now norm, 121–122
Heterogeneous groups, 129
Holistic health movement, 43
Homogeneous groups, 128–129
Hope instillation through group process,
113
Humanistic counseling
for communication disorders, 14–15
compared with other counseling
theories, 28
description of, 13–14
limitations of, 15
training in, 170
Humanistic credo, 13
Humility of professionals, 107–108

Identity
in counseling relationship, 43–44

identity versus role confusion in
Erikson life cycle, 33–34
IEP, 76, 176, 178
If You Meet the Buddha on the Road Kill Him!
(Kopp), 13
Inadequacy, feelings of, 50–53
Individual educational plan (IEP), 76,
176, 178
Industry
in counseling relationship, 41–42
industry versus inferiority in Erikson
life cycle, 33, 36
Inferiority, industry versus, 33, 36
Informing
content response as counseling
technique, 89
as counseling, 1–3, 61–62
through group process, 113–114
of parents during diagnostic process,
80–81
Initiative
in counseling relationship, 40–41
initiative versus guilt in Erikson life
cycle, 33, 36
Initiative norm, 119–120
Institution-centered diagnosis, 75–77
Institutionalization decision, 150
Integration stage of coping process, 70
Integrity
in counseling relationship, 45–46
ego integrity versus despair, 35
Interactional norm, 119
Internal locus of control, 100–102, 173
Interpersonal skills
through group process, 114
training in, 170–171
Intimacy
in counseling relationship, 44–45
in families, 160
intimacy versus isolation in Erikson life
cycle, 34–35
Irrational ideas, 25, 26, 27
Isolation, intimacy versus, 34–35
Itinerant therapy programs, 41–42

Language changing, 101–102
Laryngectomized patients, 120, 135

Leadership in groups, 117–118
Learning, approaches to, 41–43
Lecture, 41
Letting go, 165
Life cycle. *See* Erikson life cycle
Limits of counseling, 177–178
Listening
counseling by listening and valuing,
5–7, 109–110
empathic listening, 14, 91
importance of, 109–110
trust and nonjudgmental listening, 38
Locus of control, 99–102, 173
Locus of Control of Behavior Scale, 100
Loneliness, and existentialism, 19, 22–23
Loss. *See* Grief
Love, and existentialism, 19

Meaninglessness, and existentialism, 20,
23–24
Medical model
of counseling, 1–2
of diagnostic process, 75–77
Mental retardation. *See* Developmental delay
Minnesota Multiphasic Personality
Inventory (MMPI), 168, 169
Miracle Worker, The, 51–52, 53
Mistakes of professionals, 108–109
Mistrust, trust versus, 32, 36
MMPI, 168, 169
Models as clinical tools, 46
Modification strategy, in coping process,
72
Mothers. *See also* Parents
employment of, 142
guilt of, 57–58
self-esteem of, 162–163
Mourning. *See* Grief
Multiculturalism, 85, 90, 176–177
Multiple sclerosis, 66

Near-death experiences, 20–21
Norms of group
confrontation norm, 120–121, 124–125
establishment of, by leader, 118–123
here-and-now norm, 121–122
initiative norm, 119–120

interactional norm, 119
procedural norms, 122–123
respect for individual needs, 122
self-disclosure, 120

Optimal families, 159–161
Overprotection, 36, 58

Parents. *See also* Families
in affirmation stage of coping process,
69–70
anger of, 53–57, 143
case studies of hypothetical families,
95–99
communication about feelings
between, 143–144
as component in families, 139–147
confusion of, 61–62
coping process and, 66–73
death of, 150–151
Dee's total communication program for,
4
denial by, 66–68, 77–78, 80, 143–144,
162
and diagnosis by committee, 76
with disability, 147–151
divorce of, 71
and Erikson life cycle, 36
father-child relationship, 140–142,
145–146
grief reaction of, 36, 48–50, 81, 144
guilt of, 57–59, 143, 153
inadequacy feelings of, 50–53
in integration stage of coping process,
70
involvement of, in client-centered
diagnosis, 77–85
involvement of, in school-based
language intervention program,
134–135
overprotection by, 36, 58
reactions to audiologists' counseling
skills, 2–3
resistance by, 68–69
role of, in relationship to school, 43
self-esteem of, 162–163
superdedicated parents, 58–59, 143

therapist demonstration of lessons to,
41–42
training of students for parent
programs, 64–65
and triangulation in family, 140–141
vulnerability feelings of, 59–60
Patient, connotation of term, 43
Personal growth, through group process,
117
Personal system of instruction (PSI)
course, 173
Persuasion model of counseling, 3–5, 27
Poems, 81–83, 165
Procedural norms in groups, 122–123
Professionals. *See also* Audiologists;
Speech pathologists
anger of, 63
burnout in, 169, 173–175
congruence of, 14, 178
emotions of, 62–64, 105–106
guilt of, 63
humility of, 107–108
mistakes of, 108–109
as rescuers, 21–22, 51–53, 169, 177
as role-bound individual, 43–44
therapists as change agents, 175
training of, in counseling, 2, 167–169
vulnerability feelings of, 63
PSI course, 173

Questions
about cause of disorder, 84
counterquestions as counseling
technique, 90–91
of parents in diagnostic process, 80–81,
83–84
sample client questions, 94–95
"Why me?" question, 23–24, 92,
163–164

Rational-emotive therapies, 24–27, 101
Reflective listening, 14
Reflective silence, 104
Reframing
as counseling technique, 92–93
definition of, 72
during diagnostic process, 83–84

"It could be worse" phrase, 72
Rescue syndrome, 21–22, 51–53, 169, 177
Resistance stage of coping process, 68–69
Resistance to group process, 125–126
Respect for individual needs in groups, 122
Responses of counselor
    affect response, 91–92
    affirmation, 94–95
    content response, 89
    control via, 88–95
    counterquestions, 90–91
    reframing, 92–93
    sharing self, 93–94
    "uh huh" response, 94
Responsibility
    and existentialism, 17–19, 21–22
    and locus of control, 100–102
Road Less Traveled, The (Peck), 19
Rogerian counseling. *See* Humanistic
        counseling
Role confusion, identity versus, 33–34
Romantic love, 19
Rotter scale, 99, 173

Schizophrenia, 32
School-based counseling, 175–177
Schools for the deaf, 36
Self-actualization, 13, 14, 15, 169–170
Self-disclosure in group, 120
Self-esteem, of parents, 162–163
Self Help for the Hard of Hearing
        (SHHH), 70
Self-reports, by parents, 78–79
Setting of group, 129–130
Shame and doubt, autonomy versus,
        32–33, 36
Sharing self, as counseling technique,
        93–94
SHHH (Self Help for the Hard of
        Hearing), 70
Siblings, 154–159
Sign language, 22
Silence
    changing-topic silence, 103–104
    as counseling technique, 102–104
    embarrassed silence, 103
    reflective silence, 104

termination silence, 104
Size of group, 129
Special Children, Special Parents (Murphy),
        65
Speech pathologists. *See also* Professionals
    boundaries for counseling by, 177–178
    counseling by, 1–7
    as "rescuers," 21–22
    research needed on counseling
        effectiveness of, 3
    training in counseling for, 2, 167–173
Spouses with long-term disability,
        136–139
Stagnation, generativity versus, 35
Stress
    in marriage with spouse with chronic
        disability, 138–139
    on families with child with disability,
        146–147, 164–165
Stress reduction, 72, 73
Stroke patients, 112, 115, 134
Structured experiences, 128
Student training. *See* Training
Stuttering
    behavior modification for, 11
    cognitive therapy for, 26
    family therapy for, 133–134
    humanistic counseling for, 15
    locus of control and, 100
    responsibility assumed by stutterers, 22
Successful families, 161–165
Supervisory/teaching relationship, 171

Termination, 21, 45–46, 127
Termination silence, 104
Training
    author's initial training in counseling, 1
    for clinical competence and personal
        growth, 169–173
    in interpersonal skills, 170–171
    of speech pathologists and audiologists
        in counseling, 2, 167–169
    of students for parent programs, 64–65
Transactional analysis, 21
Triangulation in families, 140–141
Trust
    in counseling relationship, 37–38

in groups, 127
trust versus mistrust in Erikson life
cycle, 32, 36

"Uh huh" response, 94
Unattractive clients, 109

Valuing, in counseling, 5–7, 109–110
Vulnerability feelings, 59–60, 63

"Why me?" question, 23–24, 92, 163–164
Working group, 126–127

Notes

Notes